This health and fitness tracker belongs to:

My Goals....

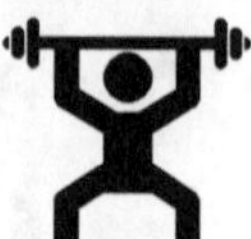

My Top 3 Long Term Goals:		Top Monthly Goals:	
Start Date		Start Date	
Accomplishment Goal Date		Accomplishment Goal Date	
1		1	
2		2	
3		3	

My WHY's....

Why #1	Why #2	Why #3

My Obstacles/Excuses....

Obstacle #1	Obstacle #2	Obstacle #3

MY PLAN when these obstacles/excuses occur:

Plan #1	Plan #2	Plan #3

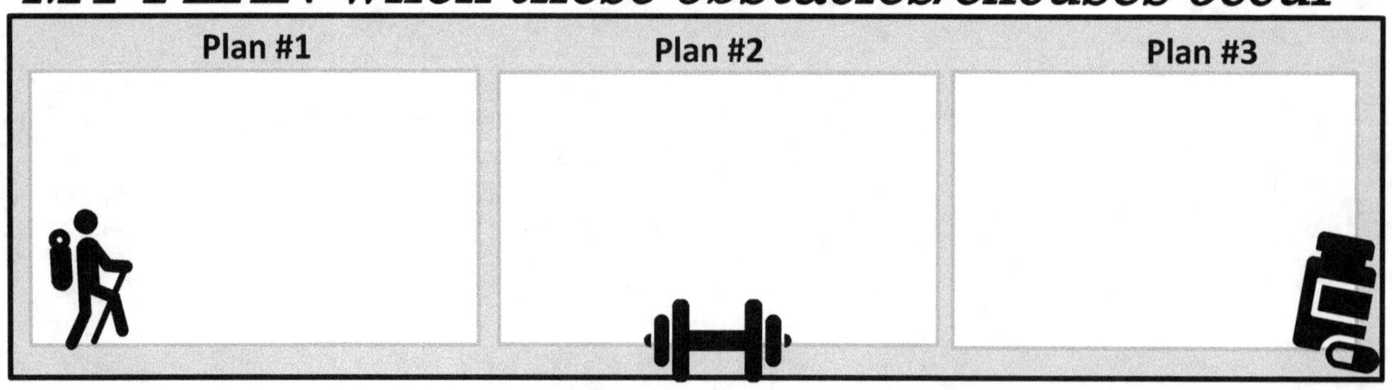

Measurements

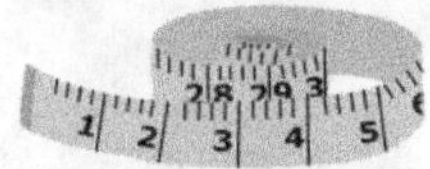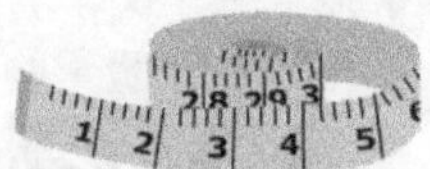

	W1	W2	W3	W4	W5	W6	W7	W8	W9	W10	W11	W12
DATE												
BUST												
Waist Above Belly Button												
Waist Below Belly Button												
Hips												
R Thigh												
L Thigh												
R Calf												
L Calf												
R Bicep												
L Bicep												
Other												

Weekly Weight Tracker

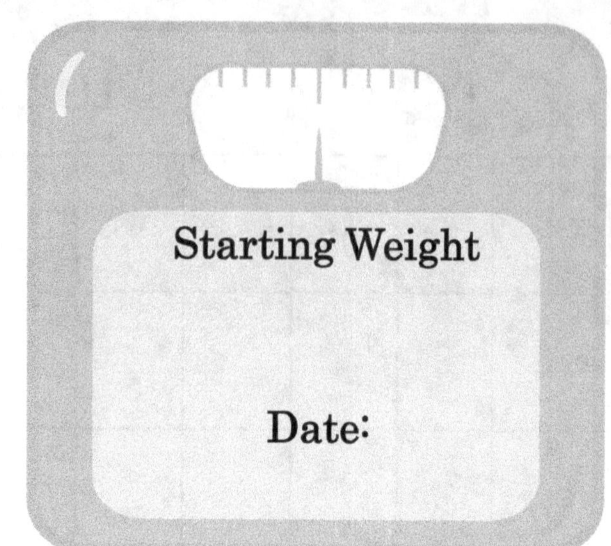

Week 1

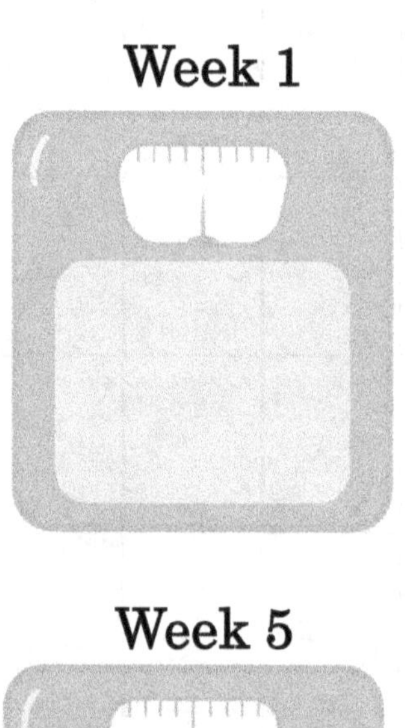

Week 2

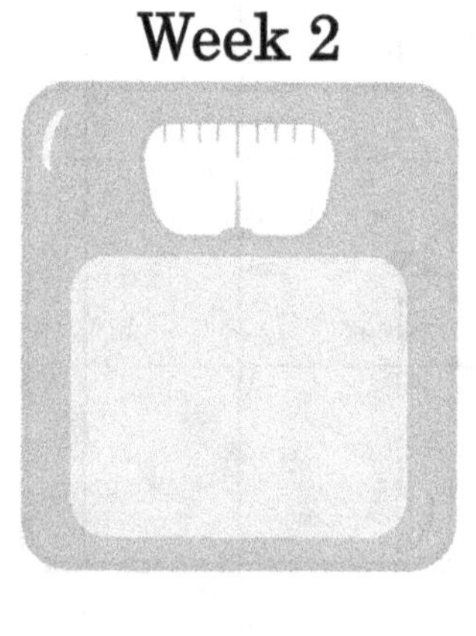

Week 3

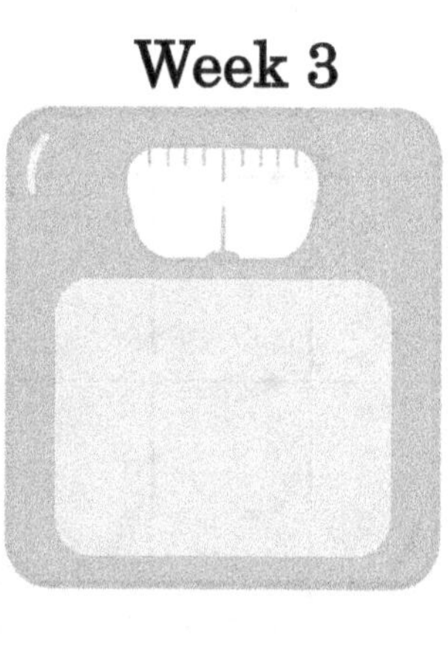

Week 4

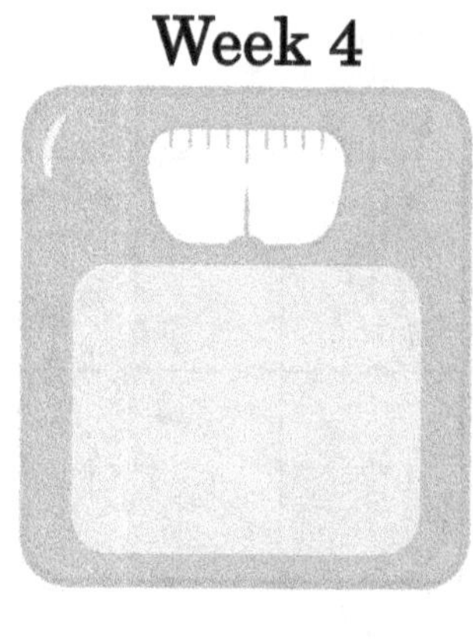

Week 5

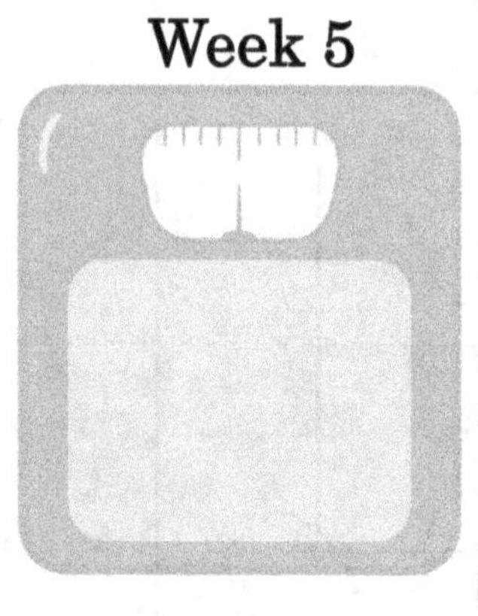

Week 6

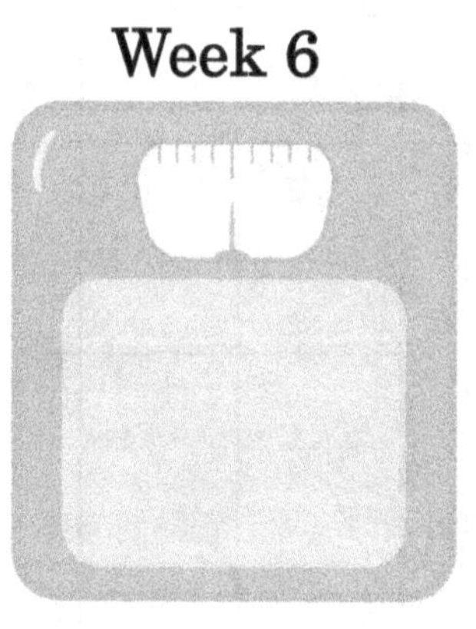

Week 7

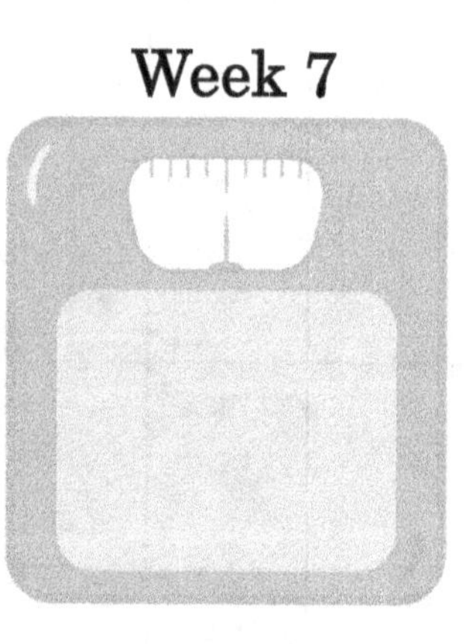

Week 8

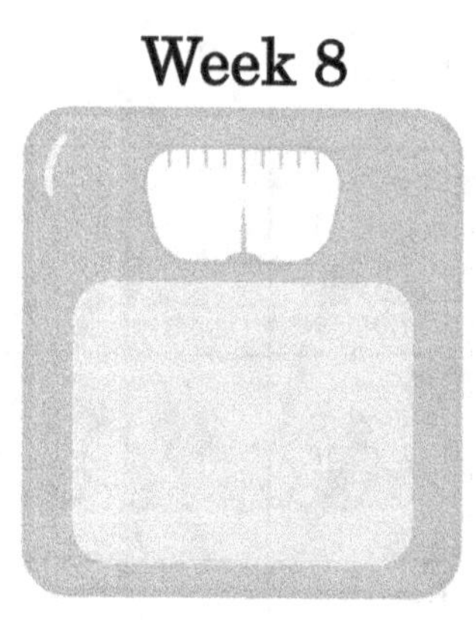

Week 9

Week 10

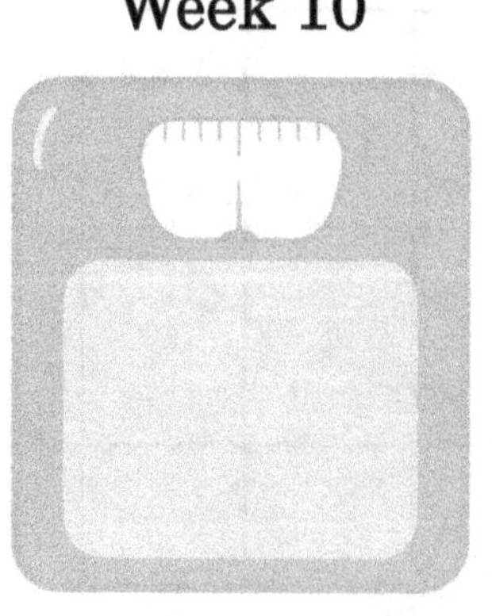

Week 11

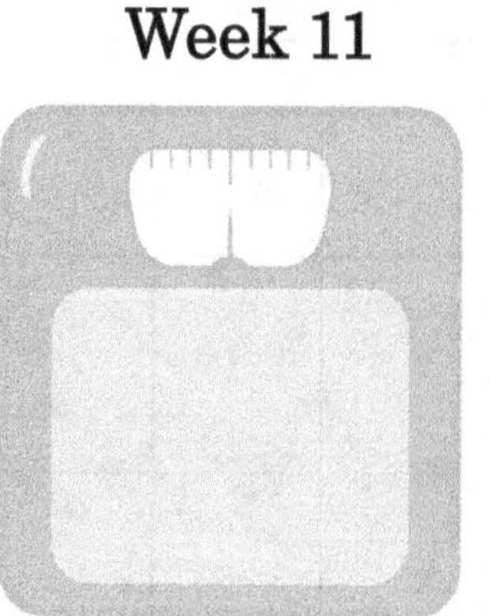

Week 12

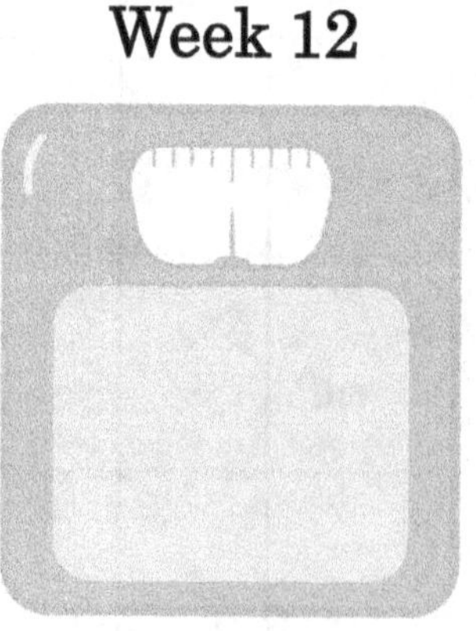

My Goals & Rewards Chart

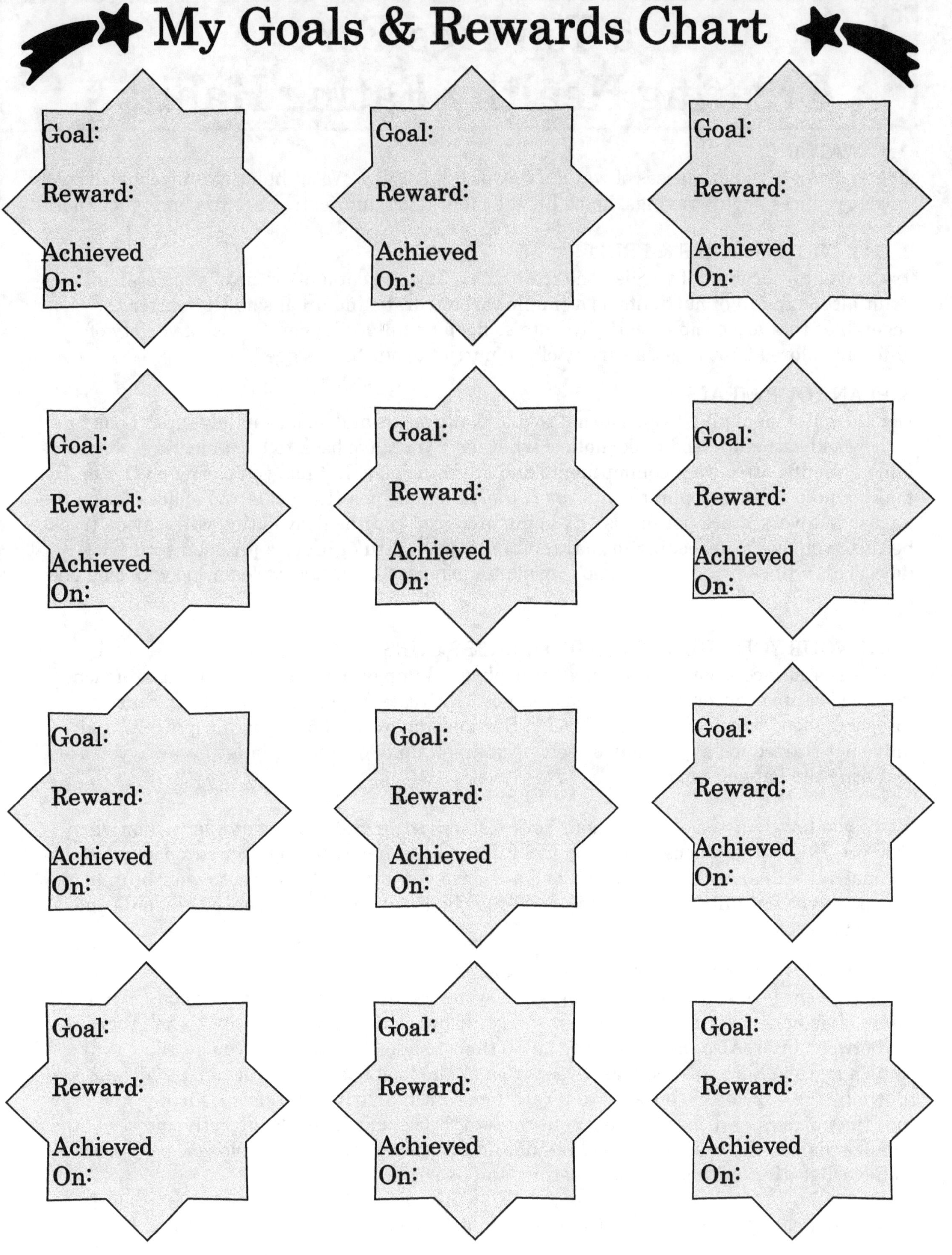

5 Top Tips For
Creating Healthy Eating Habits

1.   **WATER**

Try to drink 8-10 8oz glasses of water a day or 3-4 L a day. Water helps stabilize blood sugar levels, reduces sugar cravings, helps lift the mental fog, lubricates or joints and much more.

2. EAT YOUR VEGGIES & FRUIT

Try and eat 5 servings of veggies and fruit a day. Try and eat a 3:1 ratio of veggies: fruit. Fruit although full of nutrients is a simple carbohydrate and breaks down quicker the vegetables that are complex carbohydrate so keep us full for longer. Choose a variety of different colored fruit to get a variety of the nutrients our bodies need.

3. PLAN YOUR MEALS

Use the daily meal plan I this journal to plan your meals and snacks in advance. Look at your weekly schedule and make note of what days you have back to back meetings, doctor's appointments, after work commitments and anything else that has you eating on the go. By making note of these commitments you can plan simple healthy meals and snacks for on the go, use leftovers, crock pot meals. By being prepared your healthy eating will stay on track because you won't be needing to go through the drive thru or order a pizza on your busy days. This will help you stay on track , minimize mindless munching while saving you time and money.

4. HONOUR YOUR HUNGER AND FULLNESS CUES..

If this is a new concept identify what your physical hunger cues are (grumbling stomach, fatigue, waning concentration, mood changes…). Create a spectrum from 1-10. Start preparing food when you are at a level 2. Start eating by level 5. If you his a level 7 and have not started to eat you may be setting yourself up to overeat or binge because you are entering the hangry stage.

Once you have started eating honour your fullness scale. Stop eating at a level 7 or when you are 70% full. If you eat until you feel full then you have already over eaten as your stomach is still digesting and hasn't had a chance yet to send the signal to your bran to stop eating, if you eat until 70% full this gives your body to send the appropriate signals and translate them,.

5. EAT SLOWLY & FOLLOW THE 20MIN MEAL

When we eat fast or on the go our digestive system shuts down because our body is in a state of perceived stress. Slow down your eating by putting down your form and breathing in between bites. Also chew each bite 20-30 times. Make sure the food you swallow is in a mulch state . This helps the digestive system as the food has already been partially broken down by the enzymes in our saliva. It can then continue to break it down further and draw out the nutrients it needs before it continues to the next stage of the digestive process. And send signals to the brain that you are full and can stop eating. Eating slower may also relieve digestive irritability, gas, bloating, and heartburn.

For more healthy eating tips and support join my facebook page Health Wellness Fitness

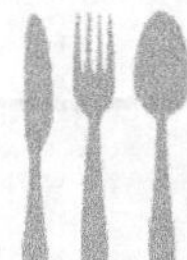 # *Some Healthier Food Choices* 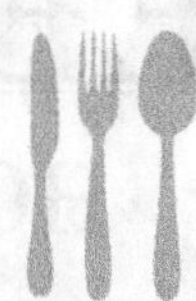

Proteins, Meats and Beans

- Beef
- Chicken
- Eggs
- Pork
- Salmon
- Shell Fish
- Tuna
- Turkey
- Wild Fish
- Wild Game

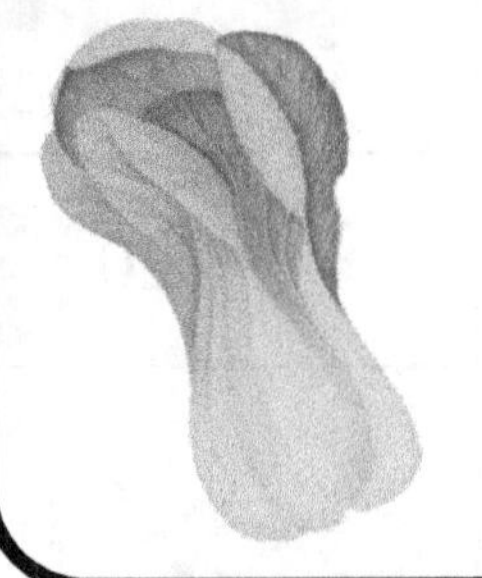

High Fibre Carbs

- Alfalfa
- Asparagus
- Beans
- Bell Peppers- Green, Orange, Red, Yellow
- Broccoli
- Brussel Sprouts
- Cabbage
- Cauliflower
- Celery
- Collard Greens
- Cucumber
- Dandelion Greens
- Eggplant
- Garlic
- Kale
- Lettuce- Butter; Iceberg; Romaine
- Mushrooms
- Onions
- Peas
- Radishes
- Red Pepper
- Spinach
- Sprouts

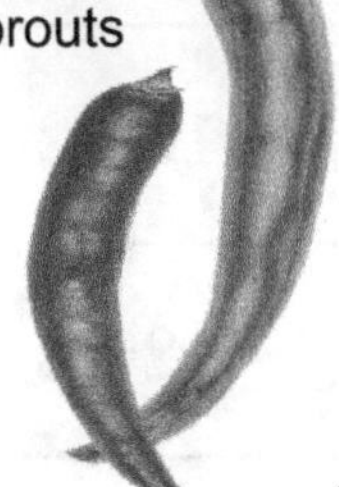

Carbs/Fibre/Fruit and Root Veggies

- Apples
- Apricots
- Beets
- Berries (all types)
- Carrots
- Cherries
- Grapes
- Lemons/Limes
- Peaches
- Pears
- Plums
- Pumpkin
- Squash- Butternut; Spaghetti
- Sweet Potatoes/Yams
- Tomato
- Watermelon
- Citrus and Tropical Fruits

Starchy Carbs

- Amaranth
- Arrowroot
- Buckwheat
- Corn
- Oats
- Quinoa
- Rice
- Rutabaga
- Turnips
- Potato

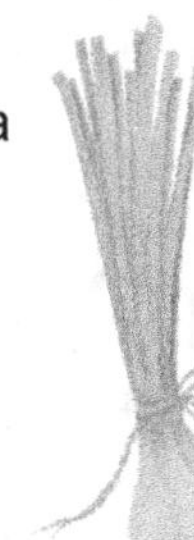

Dairy

- 2% Cottage Cheese
- Milk- Homo; Almond; Cashew; Coconut; Potato; Rice
- Greek Yogurt- Plain

Healthy Fats

- Avocado
- Avocado Oil
- Butter
- Chia
- Extra Virgin Coconut Oil
- Fish Oil
- Flax
- Flax Oil
- Ghee
- Hemp
- Nut Butters
- Nuts and Seeds
- Vegetable Oil

Spices & Seasoning

- Chili Powder
- Cinnamon
- Cumin
- Curry
- Garlic (Fresh)
- Ginger (Fresh)
- Himalayan Sea Salt
- Oregano
- Pepper
- Rosemary
- Tarragon
- Turmeric
- Vinegars

WEEK 1 FROM:_______________

HOW TO CALCULATE YOUR DAILY MACROS

Step 1-
Determine your caloric needs:
1) Weight loss
2) Weight Maintenance
3) Weight/Muscle gain

Step 2- Determine your activity level
1) Sedentary- minimal exercise or movement
2) Moderately Active- workout 3-4 times per week
3) Very Active- work out 5-7 times per week

Activity Level	Weight Loss	Weight Maintenance	Weight Muscle Gain
Sedentary/Light Activity	10-12	12-14	16-18
Moderate Activity	12-14	14-16	18-20
Vigorous Activity	14-16	16-18	20-22

Step 3- Multiply your body weight (in pounds) with your determined results from the table above from info from Step 1 &2

Example: <u>Caloric Needs-</u> Weight Loss of a <u>165lbs</u> woman
<u>Activity Level</u>: Moderately active

165 x 12 = 1980 (this would be a more aggressive weight loss strategy)
165 x 14 = 2310 (this will be a slower more manageable weight loss strategy which is advisable for maintaining long term results)

You can also choose a caloric intake in between 1980-2510. Whichever caloric intake amount you choose that is the number you will use for Steps 4-9.

Step 4- Identify your macros ratios from the diagram on the following page.

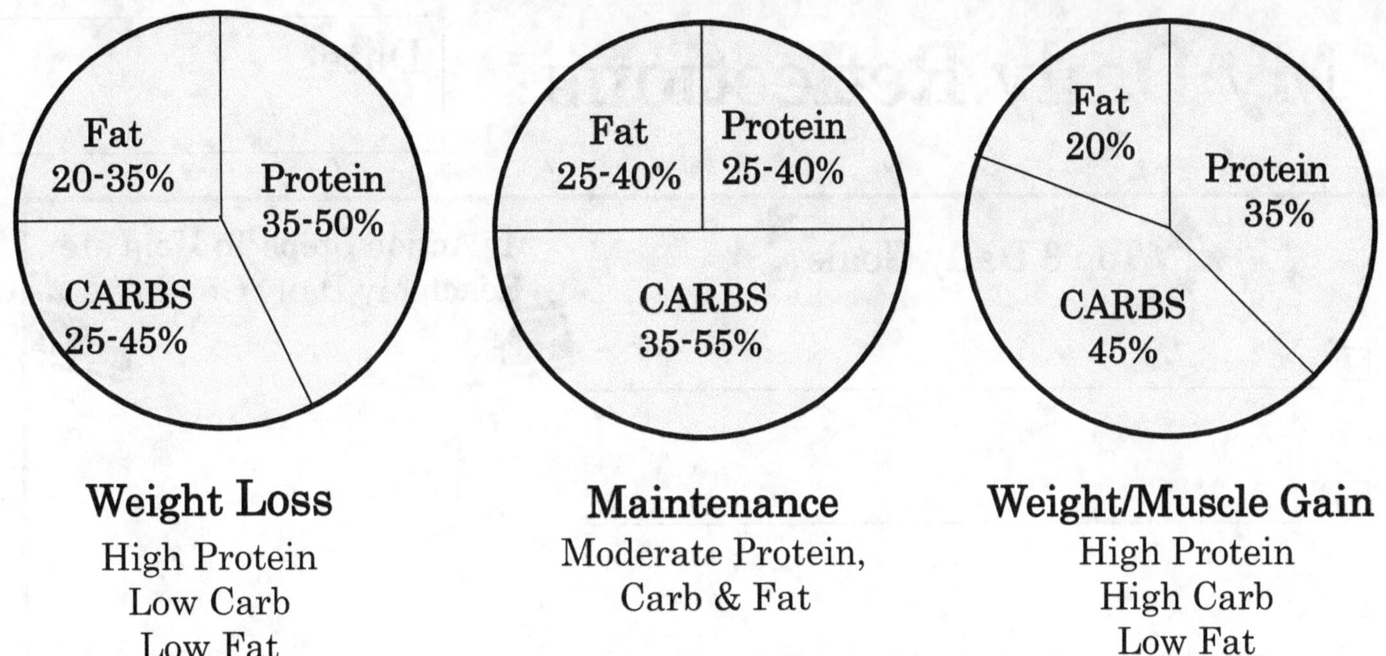

Weight Loss

High Protein
Low Carb
Low Fat

Maintenance

Moderate Protein,
Carb & Fat

Weight/Muscle Gain

High Protein
High Carb
Low Fat

Step 5- Calculate Calorie and Macros low – high ratios

Example: Using 1980 as the caloric intake here is how the low to high ratios would be calculated:

<u>LOWER End Ratio</u>
Fat= 1980 x 0.20 =396kcal
Protein= 1980 x 0.35= 693kcal
Carbs= 1980 x 0.25= 495kcal

OR

<u>HIGHER End Ratio</u>
Fat= 2310 x 0.35 = 809kcal
Protein= 2310 x 0.50= 1155kcal
Carbs= 2310 x 0.45= 1040kcal

Step 6- Convert above calories into grams

Fat= 396kcal divided by 9 = 44g
Protein= 695kcal divided by 4 = 174g
Carbs= 495kcal divided by 4 = 124g

OR

Fat= 809kcal divided by 9 = 90g
Protein= 1154kcal divided by 4 = 289g
Carbs= 1040kcal divided by 4 = 260g

Step 7- Document your daily macros based on if you use the lower or higher ends of ratios converted to grams.

Daily Caloric Intake: 1980
Fats: 44g
Protein: 1474g
Carbs: 124g

Daily Caloric Intake: 1980
Fats: 90g
Protein: 289g
Carbs: 260g

Contact Heather Marie at <u>prevailhealthcoach@gmail.com</u> if you would like assistance calculating your daily macros

My Daily Reflections

Date:

Top 3 Daily Goals

- ☐ _______________________
- ☐ _______________________
- ☐ _______________________

My Action Steps To Help Me Reach My Daily Goals Are:

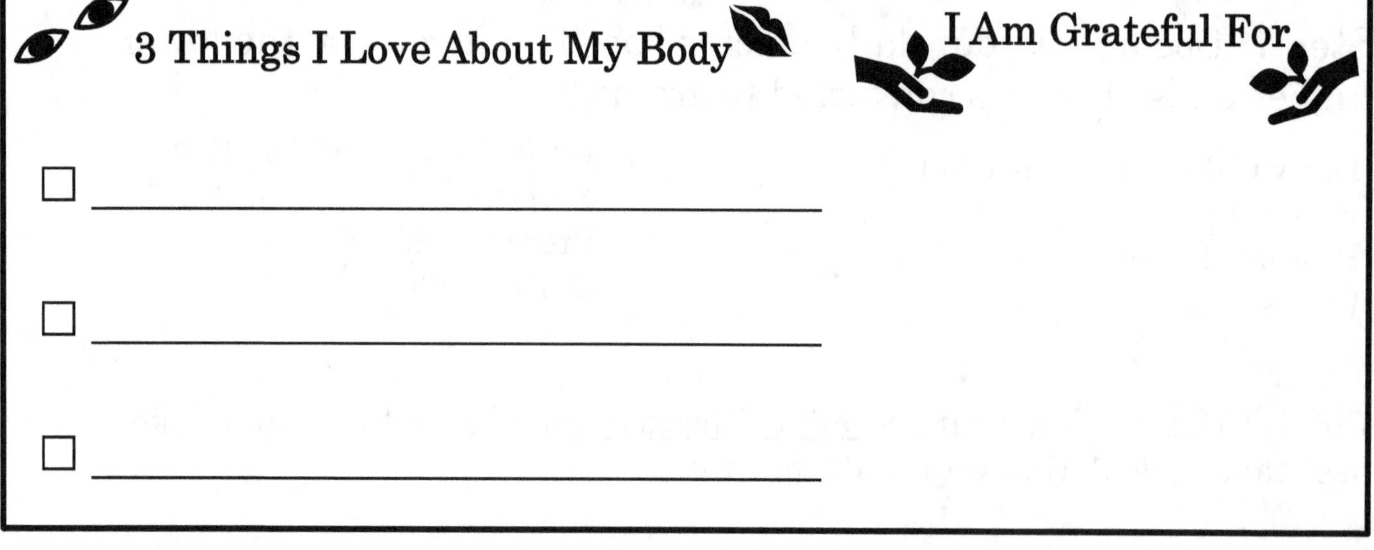

My Top 3 Strengths Are

- ☐ _______________________
- ☐ _______________________
- ☐ _______________________

Today I Found Happiness In

3 Things I Love About My Body

- ☐ _______________________
- ☐ _______________________
- ☐ _______________________

I Am Grateful For

Daily Meal Planner

MEAL PLAN		Macros Counts
Breakfast		Calories______ Carbs:______ Protein:______ Fats:______
Mid Morning		Calories______ Carbs:______ Protein:______ Fats:______
Lunch		Calories______ Carbs:______ Protein:______ Fats:______
Afternoon		Calories______ Carbs:______ Protein:______ Fats:______
Dinner		Calories______ Carbs:______ Protein:______ Fats:______

	Calories	Carbs	Protein	Fats
Calculated Macros				
Daily Totals				

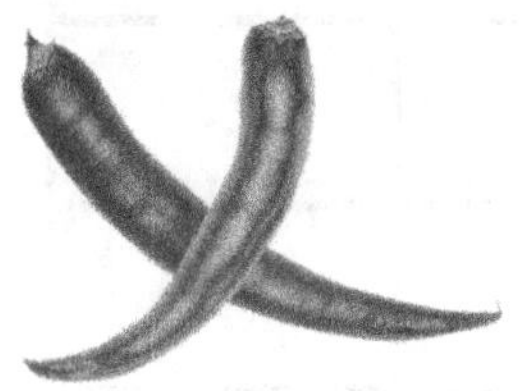
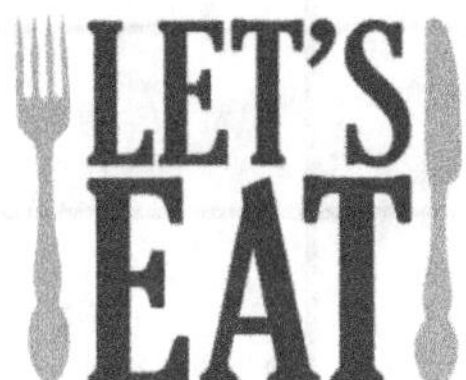

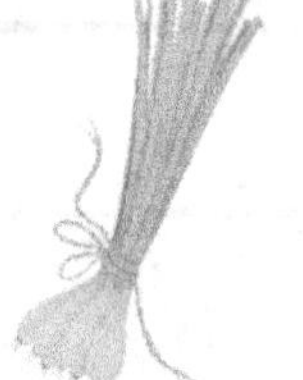

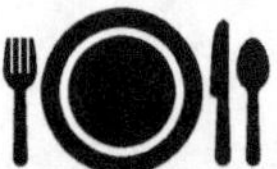 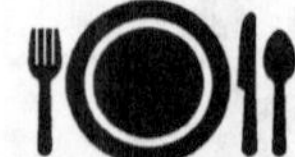

Daily Healthy Eating Habits

	Morning or Breakfast	Mid Day Or Lunch	Late Afternoon or Dinner	Evening Or Snacks
WATER- Drink 8-10 glasses or 3 L through out the day				
Veggies & Fruits- try to eat 5 servings each day				
Protein- Eat a palm size at each meal				
Healthy Fats- Eat fingertip - thumb size at each meal				
Follow Hand Portion Sizes at each meal				
Listen to Hunger & Fullness Cues				
Eat Mindfully & Slowly- Follow the 20 min meal				
Stop eating starchy carbs at 7pm				
Followed the 80/20 or 90/10 rule				
Any skipped meals				

Daily Exercise Plan

Activity	Length of W/O	Weight	Reps	Sets	Speed	Distance	Calories Burned

My Daily Reflections

Date:

Top 3 Daily Goals

- [ ] ___________________
- [ ] ___________________
- [ ] ___________________

My Action Steps To Help Me Reach My Daily Goals Are:

My Top 3 Strengths Are

- [ ] ___________________
- [ ] ___________________
- [ ] ___________________

Today I Found Happiness In

3 Things I Love About My Body

- [ ] ___________________
- [ ] ___________________
- [ ] ___________________

I Am Grateful For

Daily Meal Planner

	MEAL PLAN	Macros Counts
Breakfast		Calories________ Carbs:________ Protein:______ Fats:__________
Mid Morning		Calories________ Carbs:________ Protein:______ Fats:__________
Lunch		Calories________ Carbs:________ Protein:______ Fats:__________
Afternoon		Calories________ Carbs:________ Protein:______ Fats:__________
Dinner		Calories________ Carbs:________ Protein:______ Fats:__________

	Calories	Carbs	Protein	Fats
Calculated Macros				
Daily Totals				

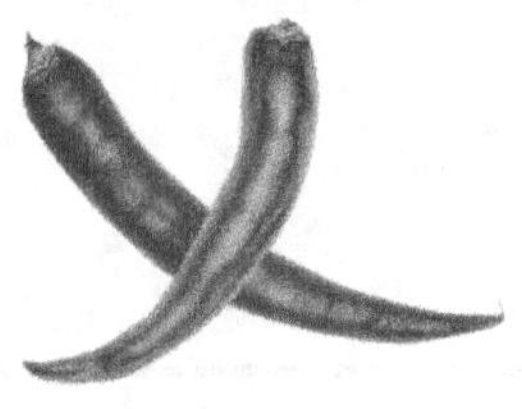
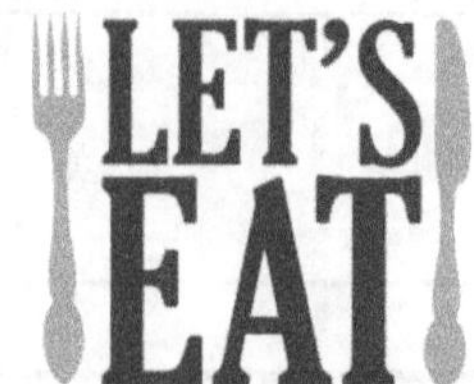

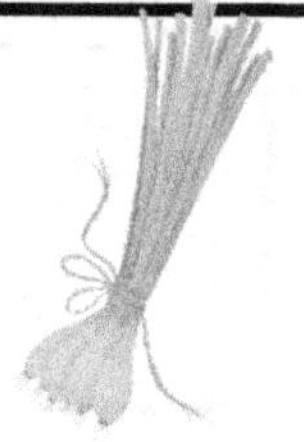

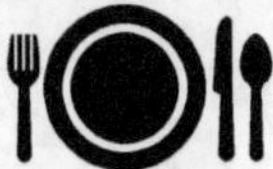 # Daily Healthy Eating Habits 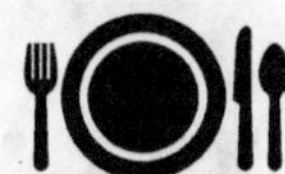

	Morning or Breakfast	Mid Day Or Lunch	Late Afternoon or Dinner	Evening Or Snacks
WATER- Drink 8-10 glasses or 3 L through out the day				
Veggies & Fruits- try to eat 5 servings each day				
Protein- Eat a palm size at each meal				
Healthy Fats- Eat fingertip - thumb size at each meal				
Follow Hand Portion Sizes at each meal				
Listen to Hunger & Fullness Cues				
Eat Mindfully & Slowly- Follow the 20 min meal				
Stop eating starchy carbs at 7pm				
Followed the 80/20 or 90/10 rule				
Any skipped meals				

ᐧᕮᐧ Daily Exercise Plan ᐧᕮᐧ

Activity	Length of W/O	Weight	Reps	Sets	Speed	Distance	Calories Burned

My Daily Reflections

Date:

⭐ Top 3 Daily Goals ⭐

☐ ___________________________

☐ ___________________________

☐ ___________________________

My Action Steps To Help Me Reach My Daily Goals Are:

♥ My Top 3 Strengths Are ♥

☐ ___________________________

☐ ___________________________

☐ ___________________________

Today I Found Happiness In

3 Things I Love About My Body

☐ ___________________________

☐ ___________________________

☐ ___________________________

I Am Grateful For

Daily Meal Planner

MEAL PLAN		Macros Counts
Breakfast		Calories________ Carbs:________ Protein:________ Fats:________
Mid Morning		Calories________ Carbs:________ Protein:________ Fats:________
Lunch		Calories________ Carbs:________ Protein:________ Fats:________
Afternoon		Calories________ Carbs:________ Protein:________ Fats:________
Dinner		Calories________ Carbs:________ Protein:________ Fats:________

	Calories	Carbs	Protein	Fats
Calculated Macros				
Daily Totals				

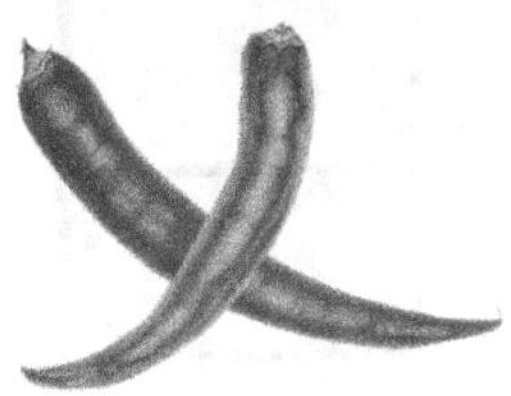
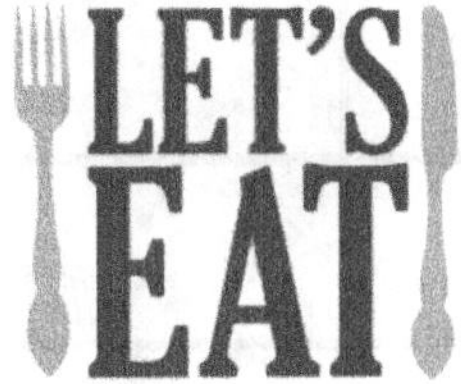

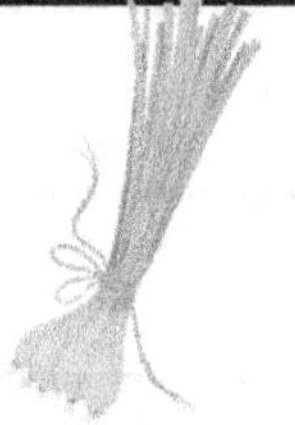

Daily Healthy Eating Habits

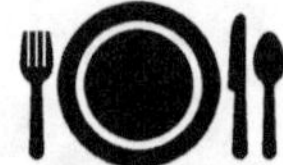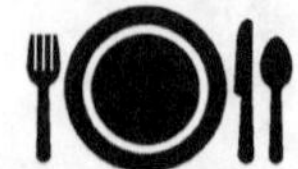

	Morning or Breakfast	Mid Day Or Lunch	Late Afternoon or Dinner	Evening Or Snacks
WATER- Drink 8-10 glasses or 3 L through out the day				
Veggies & Fruits- try to eat 5 servings each day				
Protein- Eat a palm size at each meal				
Healthy Fats- Eat fingertip - thumb size at each meal				
Follow Hand Portion Sizes at each meal				
Listen to Hunger & Fullness Cues				
Eat Mindfully & Slowly- Follow the 20 min meal				
Stop eating starchy carbs at 7pm				
Followed the 80/20 or 90/10 rule				
Any skipped meals				

Daily Exercise Plan

Activity	Length of W/O	Weight	Reps	Sets	Speed	Distance	Calories Burned

My Daily Reflections

Date:

★★ Top 3 Daily Goals ★★

My Action Steps To Help Me
Reach My Daily Goals Are:

- ☐ _______________________
- ☐ _______________________
- ☐ _______________________

♥ My Top 3 Strengths Are ♥

Today I Found Happiness In

- ☐ _______________________
- ☐ _______________________
- ☐ _______________________

3 Things I Love About My Body

I Am Grateful For

- ☐ _______________________
- ☐ _______________________
- ☐ _______________________

Daily Meal Planner

MEAL PLAN		Macros Counts
Breakfast		Calories_______ Carbs:_______ Protein:______ Fats:________
Mid Morning		Calories_______ Carbs:_______ Protein:______ Fats:________
Lunch		Calories_______ Carbs:_______ Protein:______ Fats:________
Afternoon		Calories_______ Carbs:_______ Protein:______ Fats:________
Dinner		Calories_______ Carbs:_______ Protein:______ Fats:________

	Calories	Carbs	Protein	Fats
Calculated Macros				
Daily Totals				

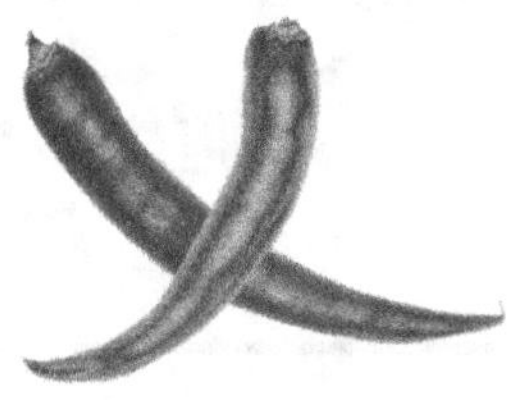

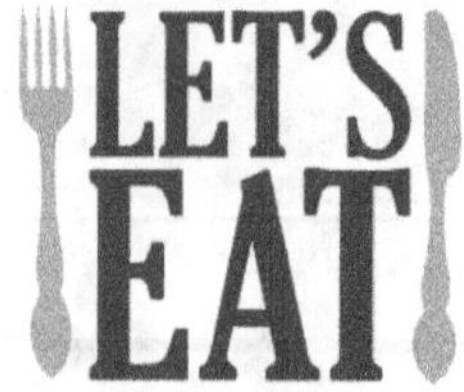

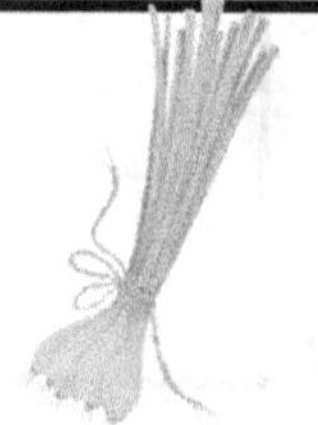

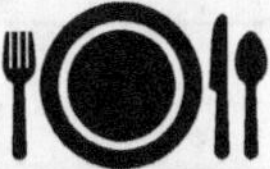 # Daily Healthy Eating Habits 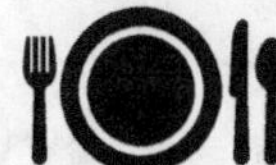

	Morning or Breakfast	Mid Day Or Lunch	Late Afternoon or Dinner	Evening Or Snacks
WATER- Drink 8-10 glasses or 3 L through out the day				
Veggies & Fruits- try to eat 5 servings each day				
Protein- Eat a palm size at each meal				
Healthy Fats- Eat fingertip - thumb size at each meal				
Follow Hand Portion Sizes at each meal				
Listen to Hunger & Fullness Cues				
Eat Mindfully & Slowly- Follow the 20 min meal				
Stop eating starchy carbs at 7pm				
Followed the 80/20 or 90/10 rule				
Any skipped meals				

Daily Exercise Plan

Activity	Length of W/O	Weight	Reps	Sets	Speed	Distance	Calories Burned

My Daily Reflections

Date:

Top 3 Daily Goals

- ☐ _______________________
- ☐ _______________________
- ☐ _______________________

My Action Steps To Help Me Reach My Daily Goals Are:

My Top 3 Strengths Are

- ☐ _______________________
- ☐ _______________________
- ☐ _______________________

Today I Found Happiness In

3 Things I Love About My Body

- ☐ _______________________
- ☐ _______________________
- ☐ _______________________

I Am Grateful For

Daily Meal Planner

MEAL PLAN		Macros Counts
Breakfast		Calories________ Carbs:________ Protein:______ Fats:__________
Mid Morning		Calories________ Carbs:________ Protein:______ Fats:__________
Lunch		Calories________ Carbs:________ Protein:______ Fats:__________
Afternoon		Calories________ Carbs:________ Protein:______ Fats:__________
Dinner		Calories________ Carbs:________ Protein:______ Fats:__________

	Calories	Carbs	Protein	Fats
Calculated Macros				
Daily Totals				

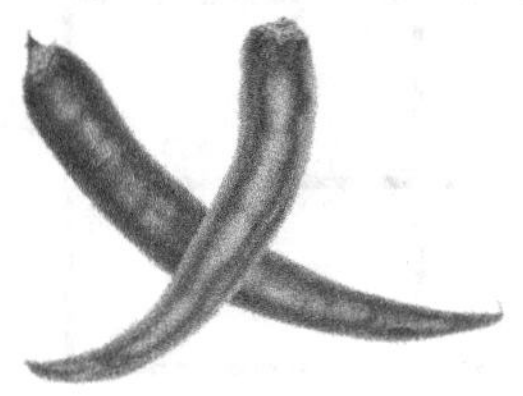

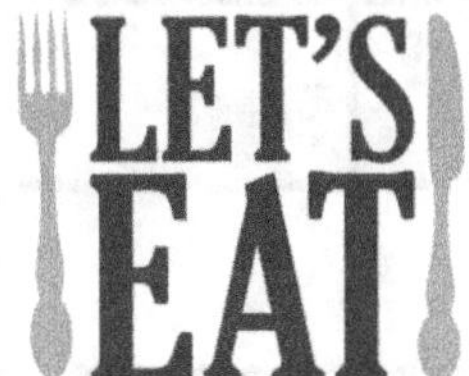

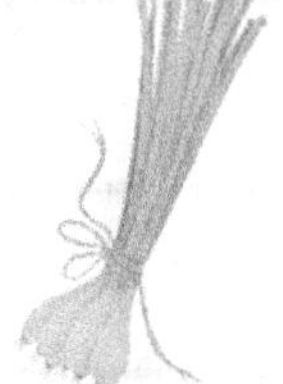

Daily Healthy Eating Habits

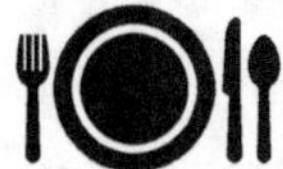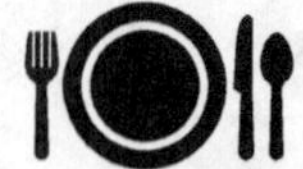

	Morning or Breakfast	Mid Day Or Lunch	Late Afternoon or Dinner	Evening Or Snacks
WATER- Drink 8-10 glasses or 3 L through out the day				
Veggies & Fruits- try to eat 5 servings each day				
Protein- Eat a palm size at each meal				
Healthy Fats- Eat fingertip - thumb size at each meal				
Follow Hand Portion Sizes at each meal				
Listen to Hunger & Fullness Cues				
Eat Mindfully & Slowly- Follow the 20 min meal				
Stop eating starchy carbs at 7pm				
Followed the 80/20 or 90/10 rule				
Any skipped meals				

Daily Exercise Plan

Activity	Length of W/O	Weight	Reps	Sets	Speed	Distance	Calories Burned

My Daily Reflections

Date:

Top 3 Daily Goals

- [ ] __________________________________

- [ ] __________________________________

- [ ] __________________________________

My Action Steps To Help Me Reach My Daily Goals Are:

My Top 3 Strengths Are

- [ ] __________________________________

- [ ] __________________________________

- [ ] __________________________________

Today I Found Happiness In

3 Things I Love About My Body

- [ ] __________________________________

- [ ] __________________________________

- [ ] __________________________________

I Am Grateful For

Daily Meal Planner

MEAL PLAN		Macros Counts
Breakfast		Calories______ Carbs:______ Protein:_____ Fats:________
Mid Morning		Calories______ Carbs:______ Protein:_____ Fats:________
Lunch		Calories______ Carbs:______ Protein:_____ Fats:________
Afternoon		Calories______ Carbs:______ Protein:_____ Fats:________
Dinner		Calories______ Carbs:______ Protein:_____ Fats:________

	Calories	Carbs	Protein	Fats
Calculated Macros				
Daily Totals				

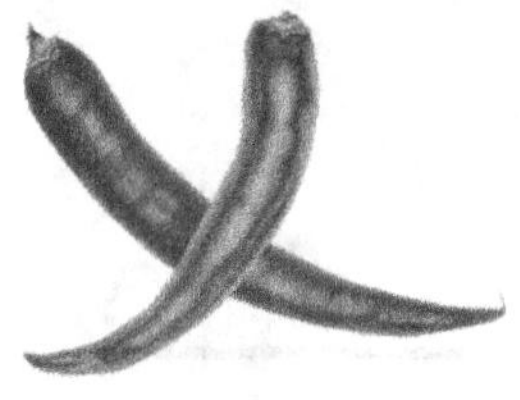
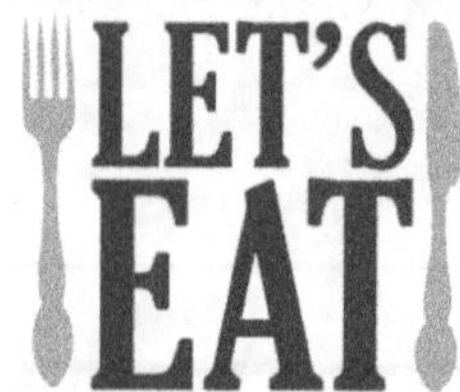

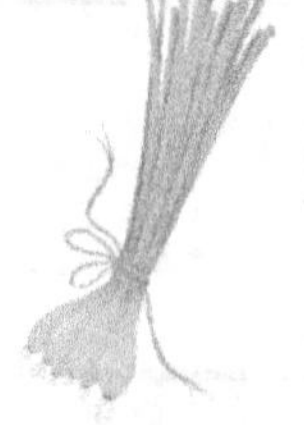

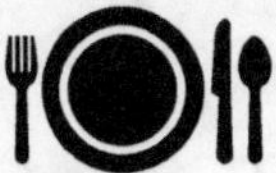 # Daily Healthy Eating Habits 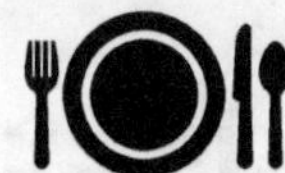

	Morning or Breakfast	Mid Day Or Lunch	Late Afternoon or Dinner	Evening Or Snacks
WATER- Drink 8-10 glasses or 3 L through out the day				
Veggies & Fruits- try to eat 5 servings each day				
Protein- Eat a palm size at each meal				
Healthy Fats- Eat fingertip - thumb size at each meal				
Follow Hand Portion Sizes at each meal				
Listen to Hunger & Fullness Cues				
Eat Mindfully & Slowly- Follow the 20 min meal				
Stop eating starchy carbs at 7pm				
Followed the 80/20 or 90/10 rule				
Any skipped meals				

Daily Exercise Plan

Activity	Length of W/O	Weight	Reps	Sets	Speed	Distance	Calories Burned

My Daily Reflections

Date:

★ Top 3 Daily Goals ★

My Action Steps To Help Me
Reach My Daily Goals Are:

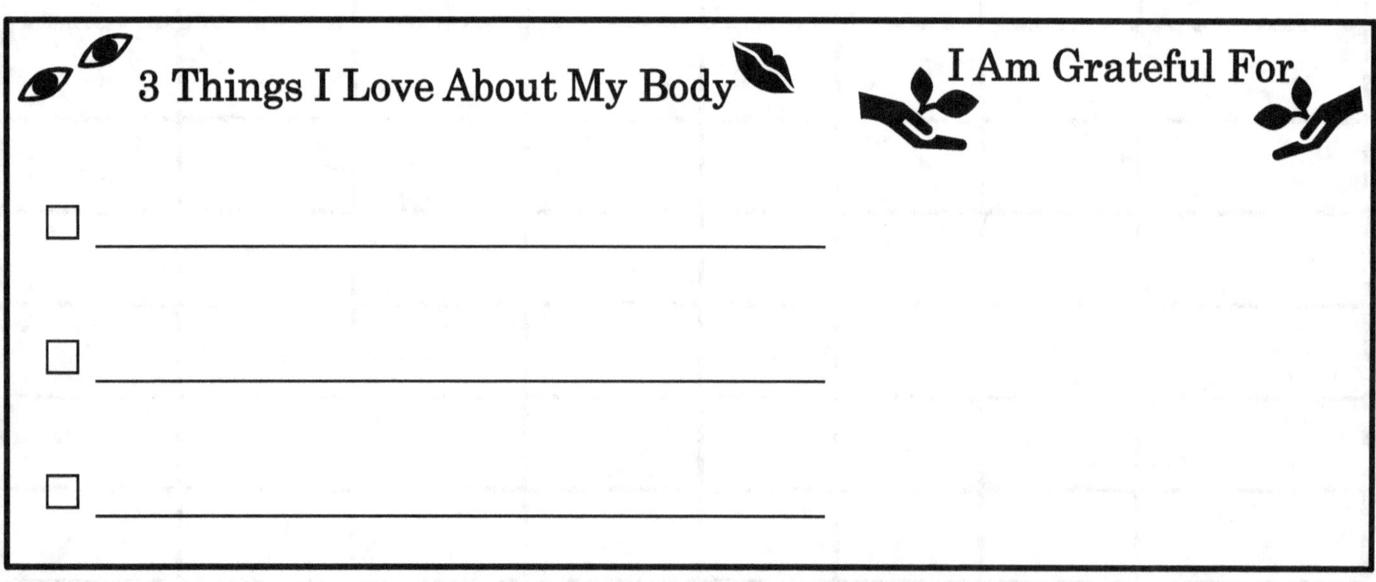

- ☐ _______________________
- ☐ _______________________
- ☐ _______________________

♥ My Top 3 Strengths Are ♥

Today I Found Happiness In

- ☐ _______________________
- ☐ _______________________
- ☐ _______________________

👁 3 Things I Love About My Body 👄

I Am Grateful For

- ☐ _______________________
- ☐ _______________________
- ☐ _______________________

Daily Meal Planner

MEAL PLAN		Macros Counts
Breakfast		Calories______ Carbs:______ Protein:______ Fats:______
Mid Morning		Calories______ Carbs:______ Protein:______ Fats:______
Lunch		Calories______ Carbs:______ Protein:______ Fats:______
Afternoon		Calories______ Carbs:______ Protein:______ Fats:______
Dinner		Calories______ Carbs:______ Protein:______ Fats:______

	Calories	Carbs	Protein	Fats
Calculated Macros				
Daily Totals				

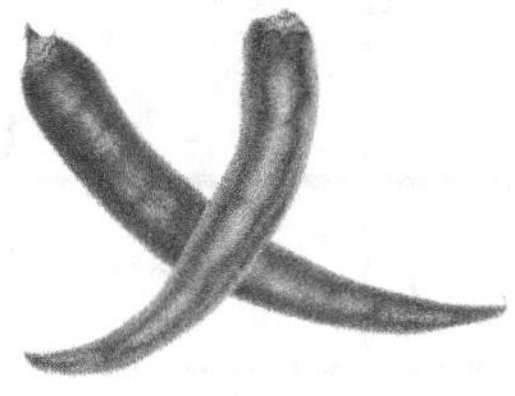
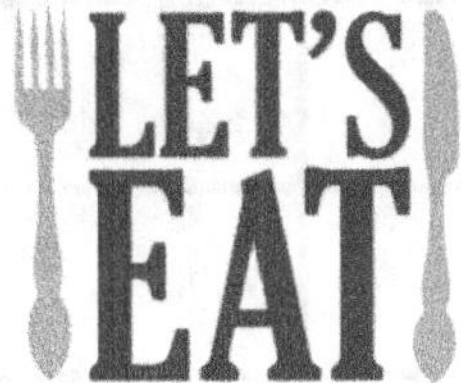

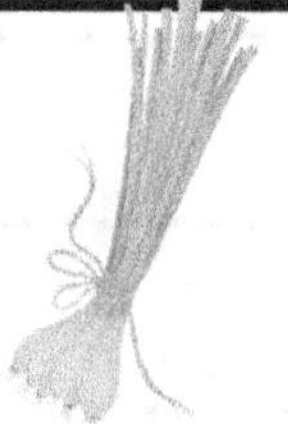

Daily Healthy Eating Habits

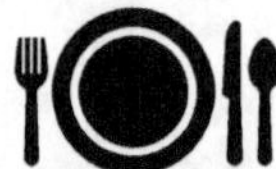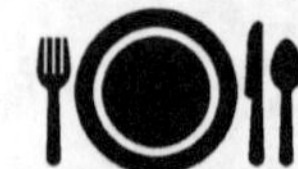

	Morning or Breakfast	Mid Day Or Lunch	Late Afternoon or Dinner	Evening Or Snacks
WATER- Drink 8-10 glasses or 3 L through out the day				
Veggies & Fruits- try to eat 5 servings each day				
Protein- Eat a palm size at each meal				
Healthy Fats- Eat fingertip - thumb size at each meal				
Follow Hand Portion Sizes at each meal				
Listen to Hunger & Fullness Cues				
Eat Mindfully & Slowly- Follow the 20 min meal				
Stop eating starchy carbs at 7pm				
Followed the 80/20 or 90/10 rule				
Any skipped meals				

Daily Exercise Plan

Activity	Length of W/O	Weight	Reps	Sets	Speed	Distance	Calories Burned

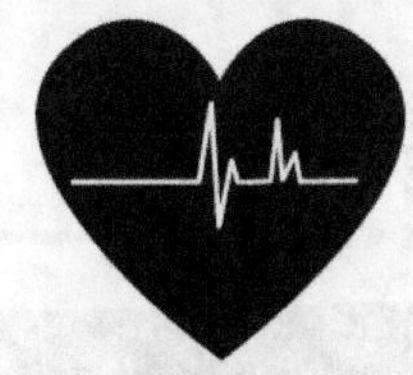

Track Your Blood Sugar

Date	Wake Up	Pre-Lunch	Afternoon	Pre-Dinner	Bedtime

Results

High					
Good					
Low					

Note Any Changes

WEEK 2 FROM: ___________

DIETARY FATS CHEAT SHEET

MONOUNSATURATED FATS

20% To 35% Of Daily Total Calories

- ✓ Olive Oil
- ✓ Canola Oil
- ✓ Peanut Oil
- ✓ Safflower Oil
- ✓ Sesame Oil
- ✓ Avocado
- ✓ Nuts
- ✓ Seeds

POLYUNSATURATED FATS

20% To 35% Of Daily Total Calories

OMEGA-3 FATTY ACIDS

- ✓ Salmon, Trout, Herring, Mackerel, Tuna, Sardines
- ✓ Soybean and Canola Oils
- ✓ Walnuts
- ✓ Flaxseed
- ✓ Beef
- ✓ Soybeans and Tofu
- ✓ Shrimp
- ✓ Brussels Sprouts
- ✓ Pacific oysters

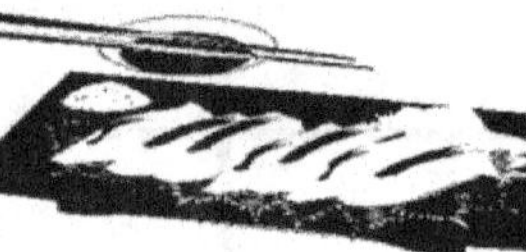

OMEGA 6 FATTY ACIDS

- ✓ Soybean oil
- ✓ Corn oil
- ✓ Safflower
- ✓ Walnuts
- ✓ Flaxseeds

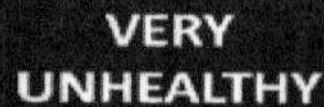

SATURATED FATS

Less Than 10% Of Daily Total Calories

- ✓ Milk
- ✓ Cheese
- ✓ Red Meat
- ✓ Poultry
- ✓ Coconut & Palm Oil
- ✓ Cocoa butter
- ✓ Processed food
- ✓ Margarine
- ✓ Cakes & Cookies

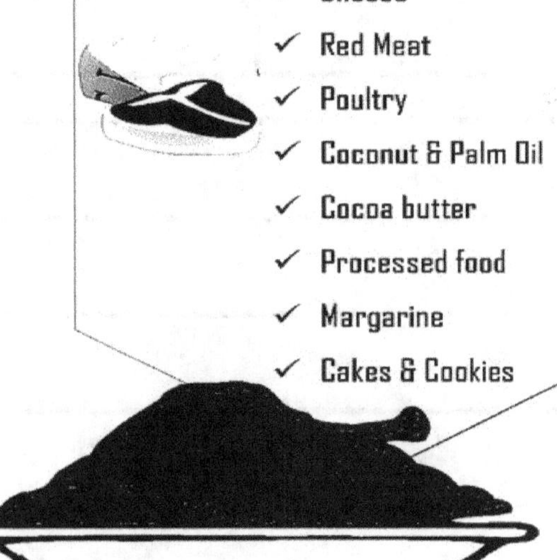

TRANS FATS

Less Than 5% Of Daily Total Calories

- ✗ Many processed foods
- ✗ Chips, and other snacks
- ✗ Commercially made cookies, cakes, and other desserts
- ✗ Lard, shortening and partially hydrogenated oils and foods made with them
- ✗ Some salad dressings

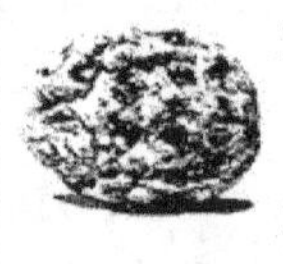

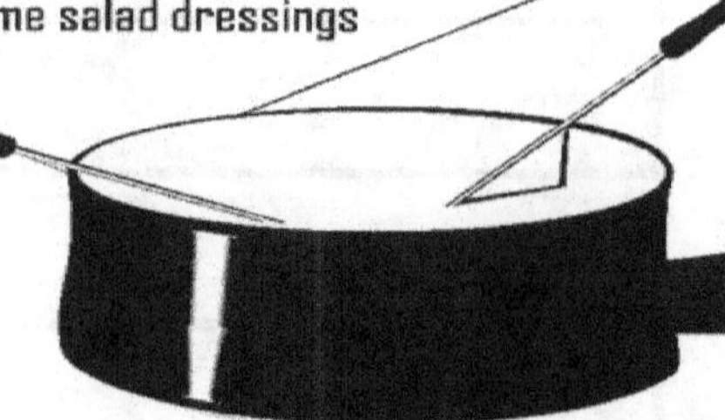
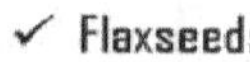

My Daily Reflections

Date:

Top 3 Daily Goals

My Action Steps To Help Me
Reach My Daily Goals Are:

My Top 3 Strengths Are

Today I Found Happiness In

3 Things I Love About My Body

I Am Grateful For

Daily Meal Planner

MEAL PLAN		Macros Counts
Breakfast		Calories________ Carbs:________ Protein:________ Fats:__________
Mid Morning		Calories________ Carbs:________ Protein:________ Fats:__________
Lunch		Calories________ Carbs:________ Protein:________ Fats:__________
Afternoon		Calories________ Carbs:________ Protein:________ Fats:__________
Dinner		Calories________ Carbs:________ Protein:________ Fats:__________

	Calories	Carbs	Protein	Fats
Calculated Macros				
Daily Totals				

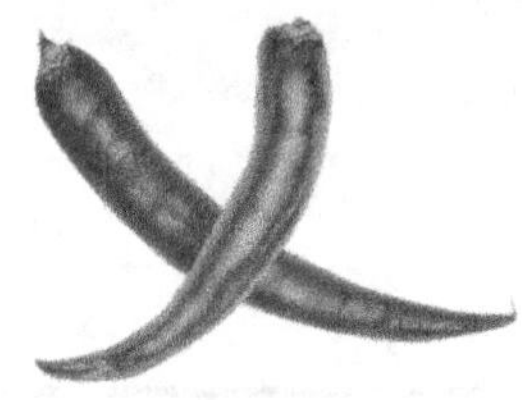
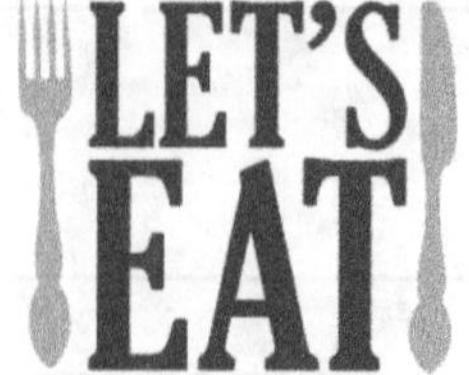

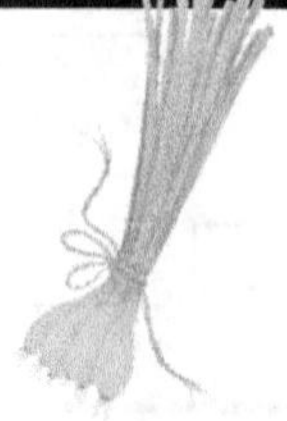

Daily Healthy Eating Habits

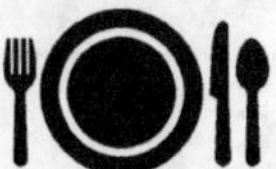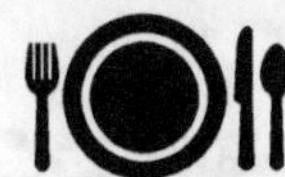

	Morning or Breakfast	Mid Day Or Lunch	Late Afternoon or Dinner	Evening Or Snacks
WATER- Drink 8-10 glasses or 3 L through out the day				
Veggies & Fruits- try to eat 5 servings each day				
Protein- Eat a palm size at each meal				
Healthy Fats- Eat fingertip - thumb size at each meal				
Follow Hand Portion Sizes at each meal				
Listen to Hunger & Fullness Cues				
Eat Mindfully & Slowly- Follow the 20 min meal				
Stop eating starchy carbs at 7pm				
Followed the 80/20 or 90/10 rule				
Any skipped meals				

Daily Exercise Plan

Activity	Length of W/O	Weight	Reps	Sets	Speed	Distance	Calories Burned

My Daily Reflections

Date:

★ Top 3 Daily Goals ★

My Action Steps To Help Me
Reach My Daily Goals Are:

- [ ] _______________
- [ ] _______________
- [ ] _______________

♥ My Top 3 Strengths Are ♥

Today I Found Happiness In

- [ ] _______________
- [ ] _______________
- [ ] _______________

3 Things I Love About My Body

I Am Grateful For

- [ ] _______________
- [ ] _______________
- [ ] _______________

Daily Meal Planner

MEAL PLAN		Macros Counts
Breakfast		Calories______ Carbs:_______ Protein:______ Fats:________
Mid Morning		Calories______ Carbs:_______ Protein:______ Fats:________
Lunch		Calories______ Carbs:_______ Protein:______ Fats:________
Afternoon		Calories______ Carbs:_______ Protein:______ Fats:________
Dinner		Calories______ Carbs:_______ Protein:______ Fats:________

	Calories	Carbs	Protein	Fats
Calculated Macros				
Daily Totals				

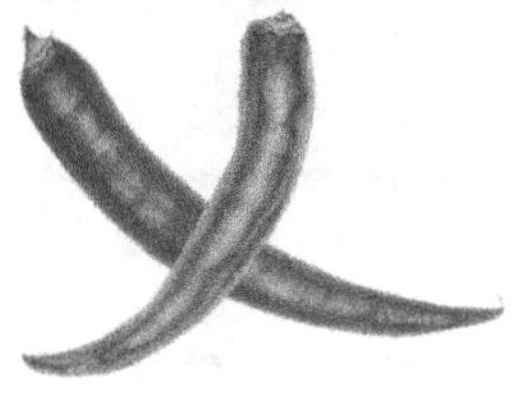
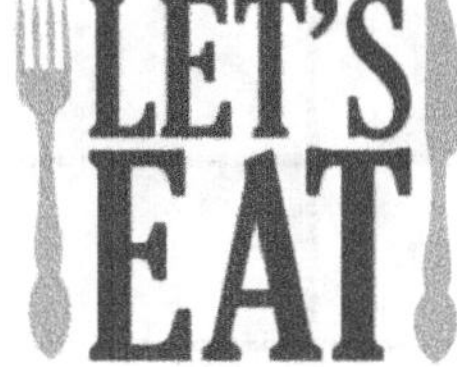

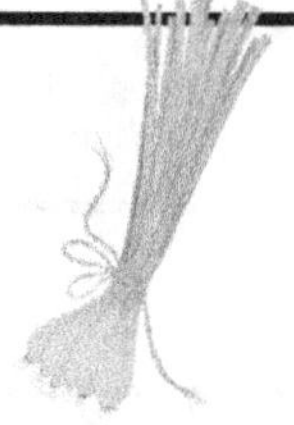

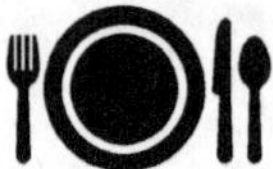 # Daily Healthy Eating Habits 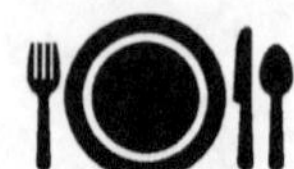

	Morning or Breakfast	Mid Day Or Lunch	Late Afternoon or Dinner	Evening Or Snacks
WATER- Drink 8-10 glasses or 3 L through out the day				
Veggies & Fruits- try to eat 5 servings each day				
Protein- Eat a palm size at each meal				
Healthy Fats- Eat fingertip - thumb size at each meal				
Follow Hand Portion Sizes at each meal				
Listen to Hunger & Fullness Cues				
Eat Mindfully & Slowly- Follow the 20 min meal				
Stop eating starchy carbs at 7pm				
Followed the 80/20 or 90/10 rule				
Any skipped meals				

Daily Exercise Plan

Activity	Length of W/O	Weight	Reps	Sets	Speed	Distance	Calories Burned

My Daily Reflections

Date:

★ Top 3 Daily Goals ★

☐ __________________________

☐ __________________________

☐ __________________________

My Action Steps To Help Me Reach My Daily Goals Are:

♥ My Top 3 Strengths Are ♥

☐ __________________________

☐ __________________________

☐ __________________________

Today I Found Happiness In

3 Things I Love About My Body

☐ __________________________

☐ __________________________

☐ __________________________

I Am Grateful For

Daily Meal Planner

MEAL PLAN		Macros Counts
Breakfast		Calories________ Carbs:________ Protein:________ Fats:__________
Mid Morning		Calories________ Carbs:________ Protein:________ Fats:__________
Lunch		Calories________ Carbs:________ Protein:________ Fats:__________
Afternoon		Calories________ Carbs:________ Protein:________ Fats:__________
Dinner		Calories________ Carbs:________ Protein:________ Fats:__________

	Calories	Carbs	Protein	Fats
Calculated Macros				
Daily Totals				

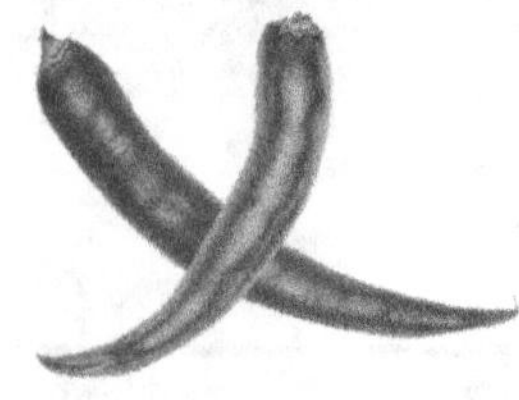

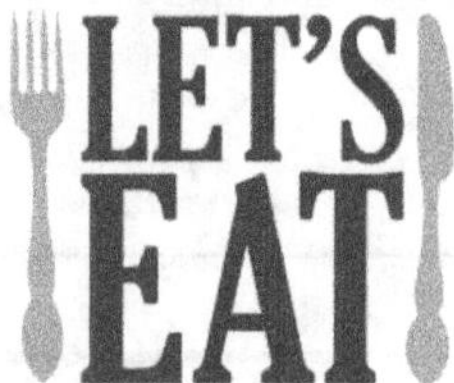

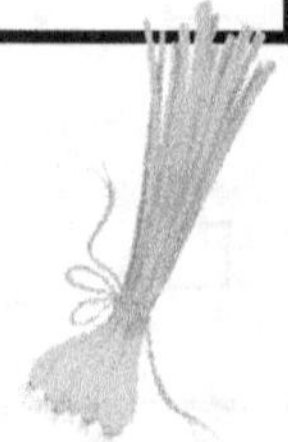

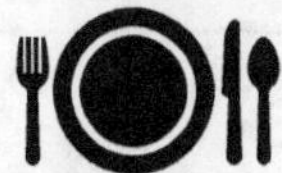 # Daily Healthy Eating Habits 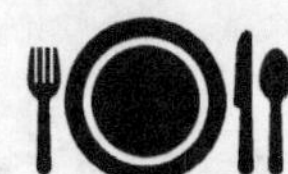

	Morning or Breakfast	Mid Day Or Lunch	Late Afternoon or Dinner	Evening Or Snacks
WATER- Drink 8-10 glasses or 3 L through out the day				
Veggies & Fruits- try to eat 5 servings each day				
Protein- Eat a palm size at each meal				
Healthy Fats- Eat fingertip - thumb size at each meal				
Follow Hand Portion Sizes at each meal				
Listen to Hunger & Fullness Cues				
Eat Mindfully & Slowly- Follow the 20 min meal				
Stop eating starchy carbs at 7pm				
Followed the 80/20 or 90/10 rule				
Any skipped meals				

Daily Exercise Plan

Activity	Length of W/O	Weight	Reps	Sets	Speed	Distance	Calories Burned

My Daily Reflections

Date:

Top 3 Daily Goals

- ☐ _______________________
- ☐ _______________________
- ☐ _______________________

My Action Steps To Help Me Reach My Daily Goals Are:

My Top 3 Strengths Are

- ☐ _______________________
- ☐ _______________________
- ☐ _______________________

Today I Found Happiness In

3 Things I Love About My Body

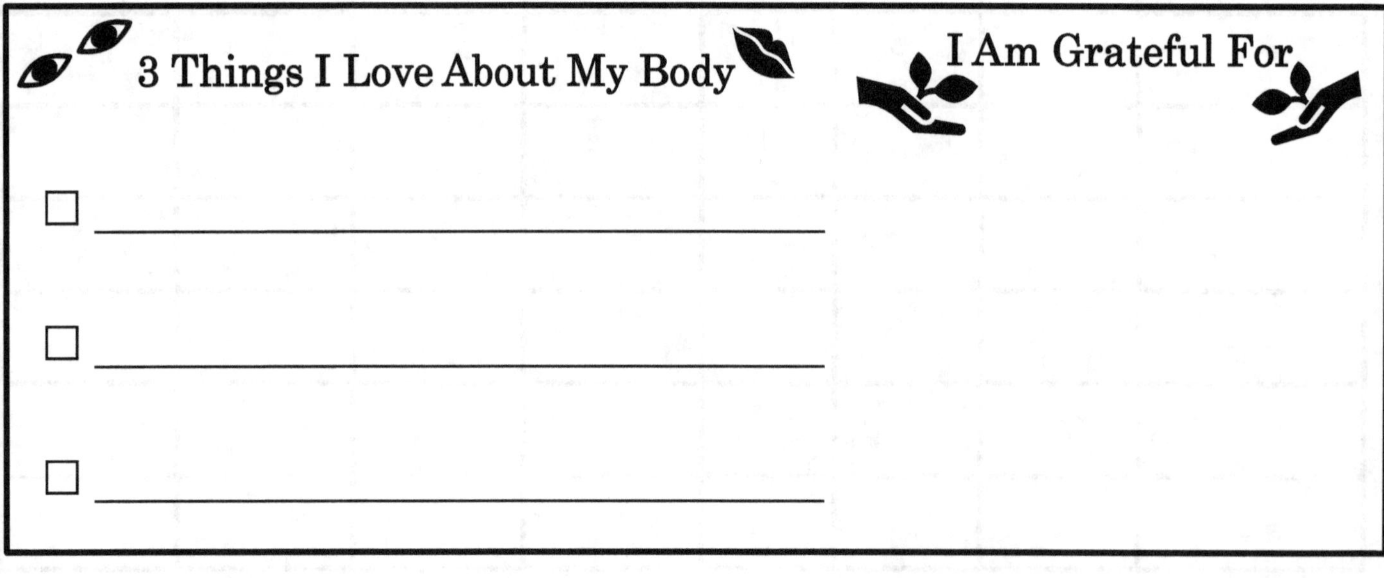

- ☐ _______________________
- ☐ _______________________
- ☐ _______________________

I Am Grateful For

Daily Meal Planner

MEAL PLAN		Macros Counts
Breakfast		Calories________ Carbs:________ Protein:________ Fats:________
Mid Morning		Calories________ Carbs:________ Protein:________ Fats:________
Lunch		Calories________ Carbs:________ Protein:________ Fats:________
Afternoon		Calories________ Carbs:________ Protein:________ Fats:________
Dinner		Calories________ Carbs:________ Protein:________ Fats:________

	Calories	Carbs	Protein	Fats
Calculated Macros				
Daily Totals				

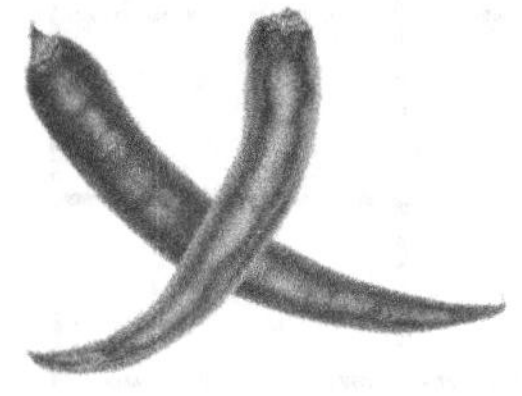

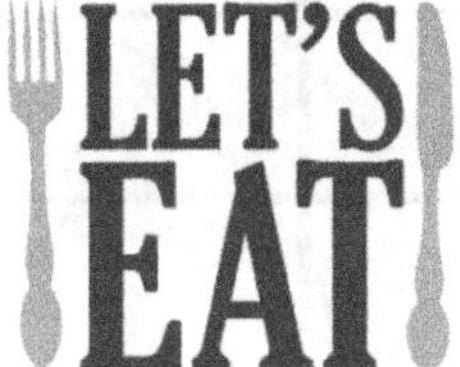

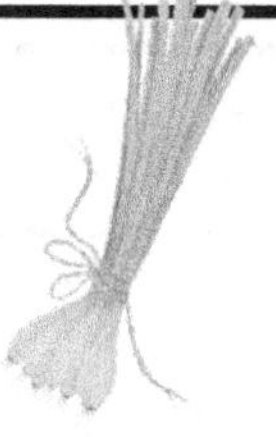

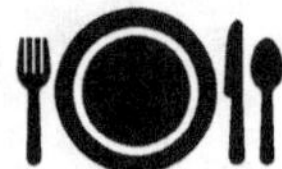 # Daily Healthy Eating Habits 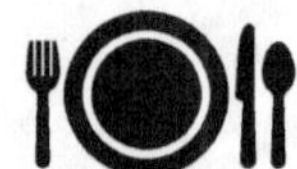

	Morning or Breakfast	Mid Day Or Lunch	Late Afternoon or Dinner	Evening Or Snacks
WATER- Drink 8-10 glasses or 3 L through out the day				
Veggies & Fruits- try to eat 5 servings each day				
Protein- Eat a palm size at each meal				
Healthy Fats- Eat fingertip - thumb size at each meal				
Follow Hand Portion Sizes at each meal				
Listen to Hunger & Fullness Cues				
Eat Mindfully & Slowly- Follow the 20 min meal				
Stop eating starchy carbs at 7pm				
Followed the 80/20 or 90/10 rule				
Any skipped meals				

Daily Exercise Plan

Activity	Length of W/O	Weight	Reps	Sets	Speed	Distance	Calories Burned

My Daily Reflections

Date:

Top 3 Daily Goals

☐ _______________________

☐ _______________________

☐ _______________________

My Action Steps To Help Me Reach My Daily Goals Are:

My Top 3 Strengths Are

☐ _______________________

☐ _______________________

☐ _______________________

Today I Found Happiness In

3 Things I Love About My Body

☐ _______________________

☐ _______________________

☐ _______________________

I Am Grateful For

Daily Meal Planner

MEAL PLAN		Macros Counts
Breakfast		Calories_______ Carbs:_______ Protein:_______ Fats:_________
Mid Morning		Calories_______ Carbs:_______ Protein:_______ Fats:_________
Lunch		Calories_______ Carbs:_______ Protein:_______ Fats:_________
Afternoon		Calories_______ Carbs:_______ Protein:_______ Fats:_________
Dinner		Calories_______ Carbs:_______ Protein:_______ Fats:_________

	Calories	Carbs	Protein	Fats
Calculated Macros				
Daily Totals				

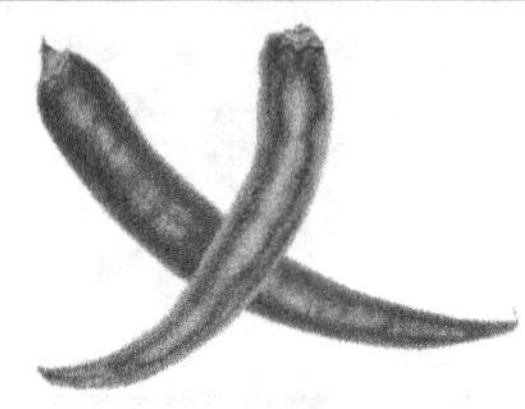
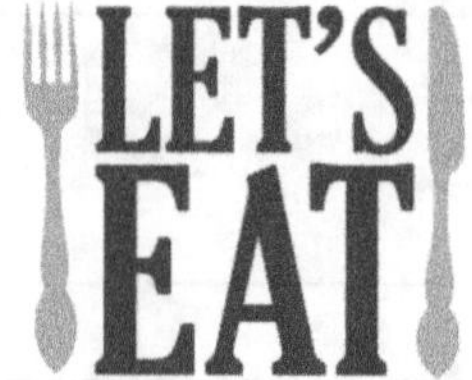

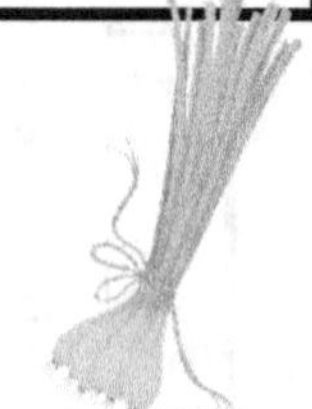

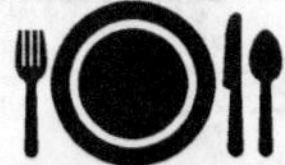 # Daily Healthy Eating Habits 

	Morning or Breakfast	Mid Day Or Lunch	Late Afternoon or Dinner	Evening Or Snacks
WATER- Drink 8-10 glasses or 3 L through out the day				
Veggies & Fruits- try to eat 5 servings each day				
Protein- Eat a palm size at each meal				
Healthy Fats- Eat fingertip - thumb size at each meal				
Follow Hand Portion Sizes at each meal				
Listen to Hunger & Fullness Cues				
Eat Mindfully & Slowly- Follow the 20 min meal				
Stop eating starchy carbs at 7pm				
Followed the 80/20 or 90/10 rule				
Any skipped meals				

Daily Exercise Plan

Activity	Length of W/O	Weight	Reps	Sets	Speed	Distance	Calories Burned

My Daily Reflections

Date:

Top 3 Daily Goals

My Action Steps To Help Me Reach My Daily Goals Are:

- [ ] ______________________
- [ ] ______________________
- [ ] ______________________

My Top 3 Strengths Are

Today I Found Happiness In

- [ ] ______________________
- [ ] ______________________
- [ ] ______________________

3 Things I Love About My Body

I Am Grateful For

- [ ] ______________________
- [ ] ______________________
- [ ] ______________________

Daily Meal Planner

MEAL PLAN		Macros Counts
Breakfast		Calories________ Carbs:________ Protein:______ Fats:________
Mid Morning		Calories________ Carbs:________ Protein:______ Fats:________
Lunch		Calories________ Carbs:________ Protein:______ Fats:________
Afternoon		Calories________ Carbs:________ Protein:______ Fats:________
Dinner		Calories________ Carbs:________ Protein:______ Fats:________

	Calories	Carbs	Protein	Fats
Calculated Macros				
Daily Totals				

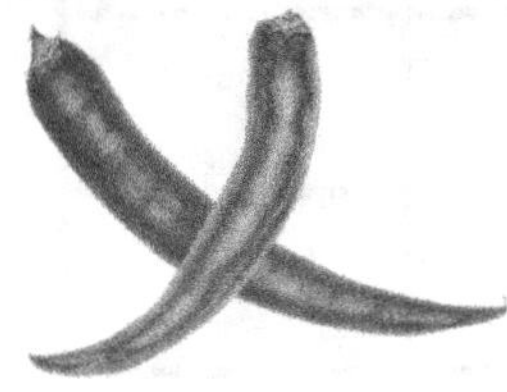
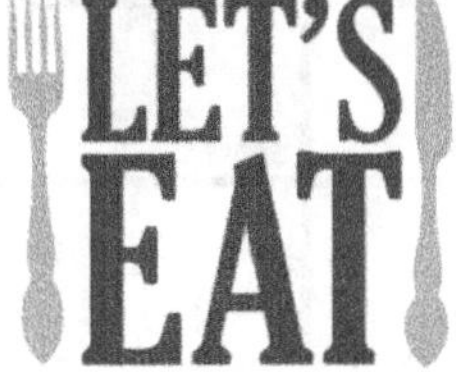

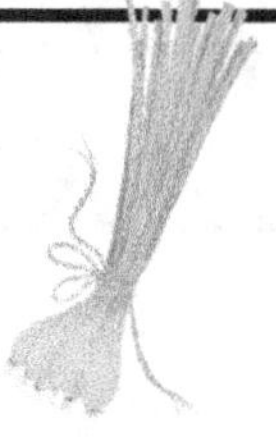

Daily Healthy Eating Habits

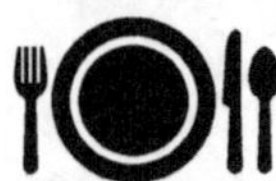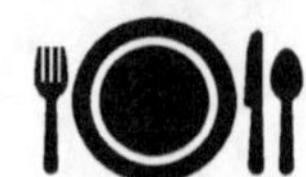

	Morning or Breakfast	Mid Day Or Lunch	Late Afternoon or Dinner	Evening Or Snacks
WATER- Drink 8-10 glasses or 3 L through out the day				
Veggies & Fruits- try to eat 5 servings each day				
Protein- Eat a palm size at each meal				
Healthy Fats- Eat fingertip - thumb size at each meal				
Follow Hand Portion Sizes at each meal				
Listen to Hunger & Fullness Cues				
Eat Mindfully & Slowly- Follow the 20 min meal				
Stop eating starchy carbs at 7pm				
Followed the 80/20 or 90/10 rule				
Any skipped meals				

Daily Exercise Plan

Activity	Length of W/O	Weight	Reps	Sets	Speed	Distance	Calories Burned

My Daily Reflections

Date:

★ Top 3 Daily Goals ★

My Action Steps To Help Me Reach My Daily Goals Are:

- ☐ _______________________________
- ☐ _______________________________
- ☐ _______________________________

♥ My Top 3 Strengths Are ♥

Today I Found Happiness In

- ☐ _______________________________
- ☐ _______________________________
- ☐ _______________________________

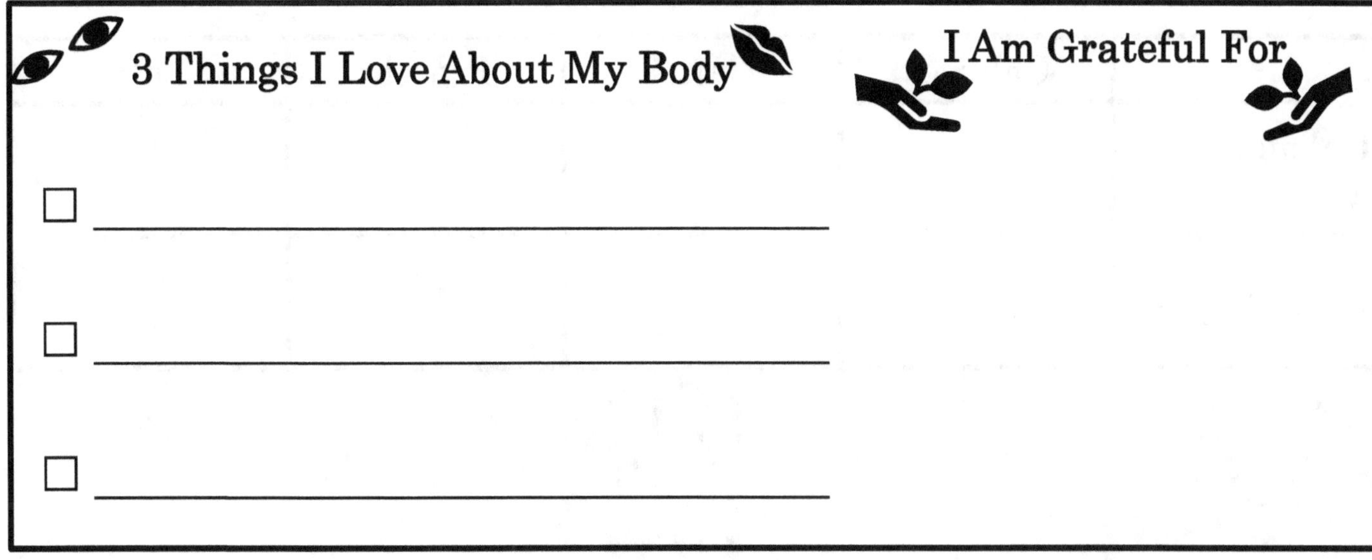

3 Things I Love About My Body

I Am Grateful For

- ☐ _______________________________
- ☐ _______________________________
- ☐ _______________________________

Daily Meal Planner

MEAL PLAN		Macros Counts
Breakfast		Calories________ Carbs:________ Protein:________ Fats:__________
Mid Morning		Calories________ Carbs:________ Protein:________ Fats:__________
Lunch		Calories________ Carbs:________ Protein:________ Fats:__________
Afternoon		Calories________ Carbs:________ Protein:________ Fats:__________
Dinner		Calories________ Carbs:________ Protein:________ Fats:__________

	Calories	Carbs	Protein	Fats
Calculated Macros				
Daily Totals				

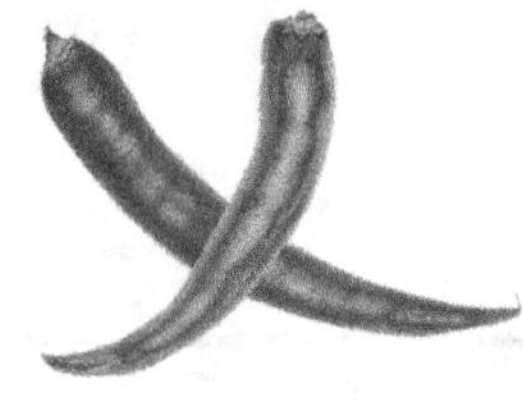
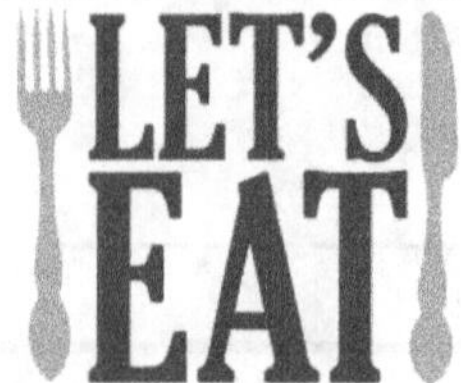

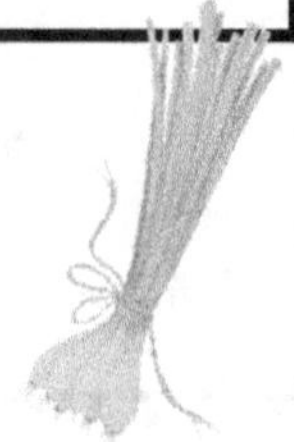

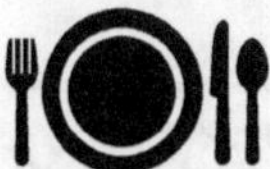 # Daily Healthy Eating Habits 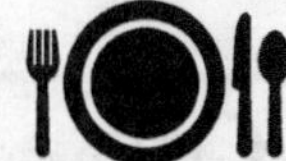

	Morning or Breakfast	Mid Day Or Lunch	Late Afternoon or Dinner	Evening Or Snacks
WATER- Drink 8-10 glasses or 3 L through out the day				
Veggies & Fruits- try to eat 5 servings each day				
Protein- Eat a palm size at each meal				
Healthy Fats- Eat fingertip - thumb size at each meal				
Follow Hand Portion Sizes at each meal				
Listen to Hunger & Fullness Cues				
Eat Mindfully & Slowly- Follow the 20 min meal				
Stop eating starchy carbs at 7pm				
Followed the 80/20 or 90/10 rule				
Any skipped meals				

Daily Exercise Plan

Activity	Length of W/O	Weight	Reps	Sets	Speed	Distance	Calories Burned

<table>
<tr><td>Week Of:</td><td colspan="2">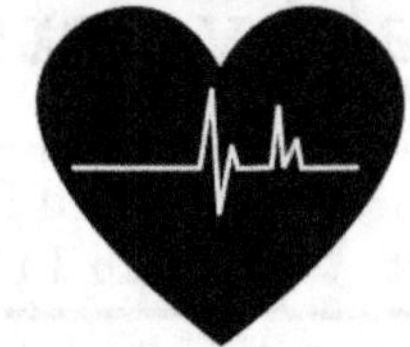</td><td colspan="3">Track Your Blood Sugar</td></tr>
</table>

Date	Wake Up	Pre-Lunch	Afternoon	Pre-Dinner	Bedtime

Results

High					
Good					
Low					

Note Any Changes

WEEK 3 FROM:_______________
START
PROUDLY
BEING
YOURSELF

My Daily Reflections

Date:

Top 3 Daily Goals

My Action Steps To Help Me
Reach My Daily Goals Are:

☐ _______________________

☐ _______________________

☐ _______________________

My Top 3 Strengths Are

Today I Found Happiness In

☐ _______________________

☐ _______________________

☐ _______________________

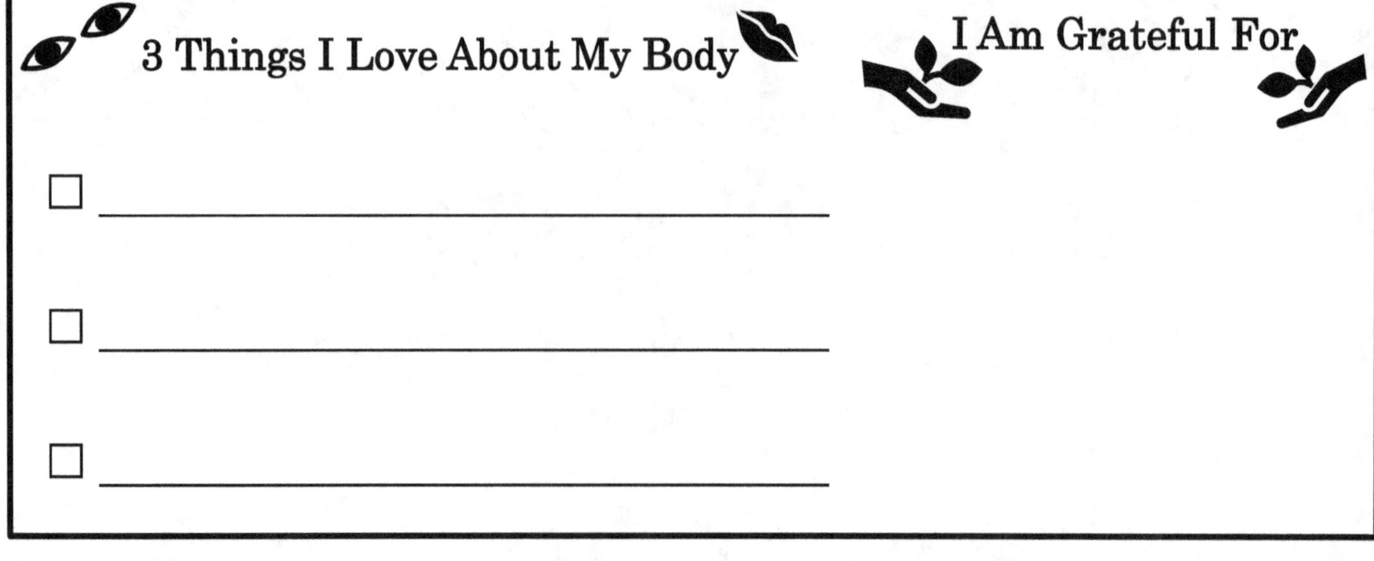

3 Things I Love About My Body

I Am Grateful For

☐ _______________________

☐ _______________________

☐ _______________________

Daily Meal Planner

MEAL PLAN		Macros Counts
Breakfast		Calories______ Carbs:______ Protein:______ Fats:________
Mid Morning		Calories______ Carbs:______ Protein:______ Fats:________
Lunch		Calories______ Carbs:______ Protein:______ Fats:________
Afternoon		Calories______ Carbs:______ Protein:______ Fats:________
Dinner		Calories______ Carbs:______ Protein:______ Fats:________

	Calories	Carbs	Protein	Fats
Calculated Macros				
Daily Totals				

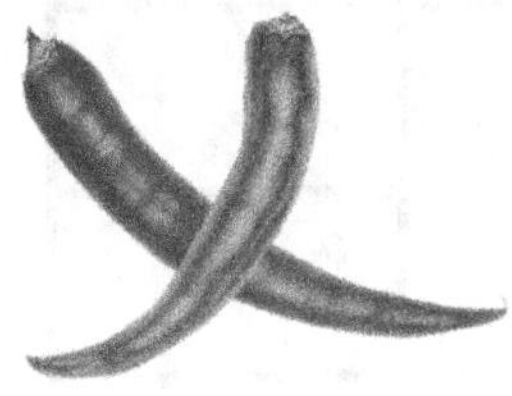

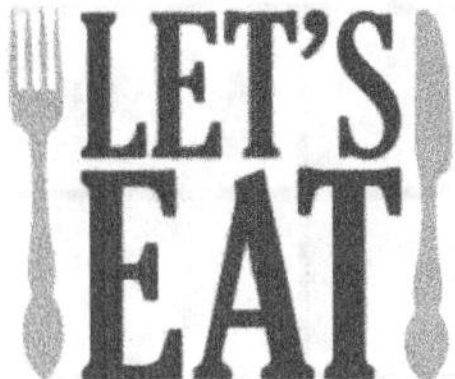

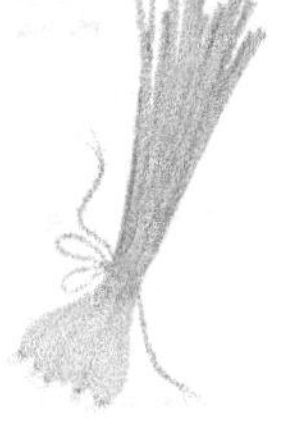

Daily Healthy Eating Habits

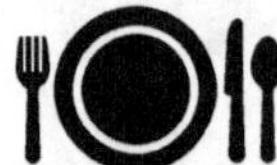
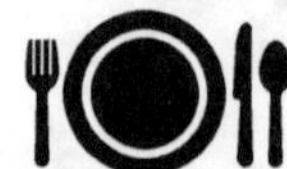

	Morning or Breakfast	Mid Day Or Lunch	Late Afternoon or Dinner	Evening Or Snacks
WATER- Drink 8-10 glasses or 3 L through out the day				
Veggies & Fruits- try to eat 5 servings each day				
Protein- Eat a palm size at each meal				
Healthy Fats- Eat fingertip - thumb size at each meal				
Follow Hand Portion Sizes at each meal				
Listen to Hunger & Fullness Cues				
Eat Mindfully & Slowly- Follow the 20 min meal				
Stop eating starchy carbs at 7pm				
Followed the 80/20 or 90/10 rule				
Any skipped meals				

Daily Exercise Plan

Activity	Length of W/O	Weight	Reps	Sets	Speed	Distance	Calories Burned

My Daily Reflections

Date:

⭐ Top 3 Daily Goals ⭐

My Action Steps To Help Me
Reach My Daily Goals Are:

- ☐ _______________________
- ☐ _______________________
- ☐ _______________________

♥ My Top 3 Strengths Are ♥

Today I Found Happiness In

- ☐ _______________________
- ☐ _______________________
- ☐ _______________________

3 Things I Love About My Body

I Am Grateful For

- ☐ _______________________
- ☐ _______________________
- ☐ _______________________

Daily Meal Planner

MEAL PLAN		Macros Counts
Breakfast		Calories______ Carbs:______ Protein:______ Fats:________
Mid Morning		Calories______ Carbs:______ Protein:______ Fats:________
Lunch		Calories______ Carbs:______ Protein:______ Fats:________
Afternoon		Calories______ Carbs:______ Protein:______ Fats:________
Dinner		Calories______ Carbs:______ Protein:______ Fats:________

	Calories	Carbs	Protein	Fats
Calculated Macros				
Daily Totals				

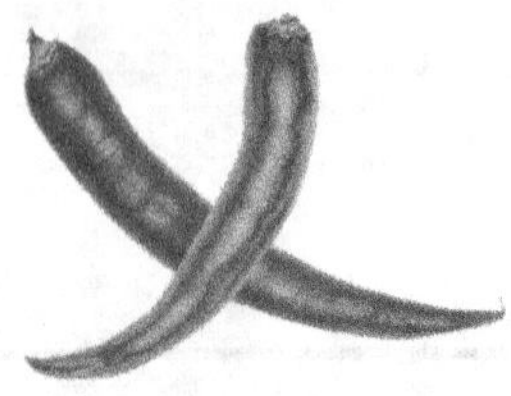
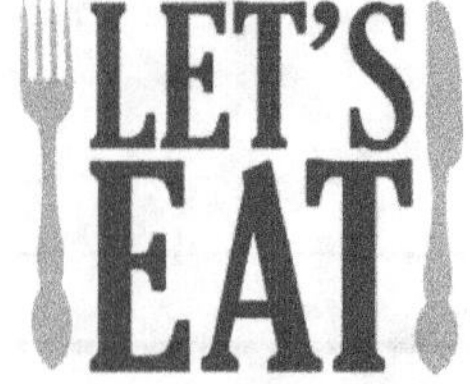

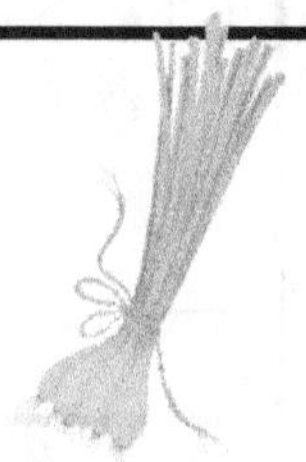

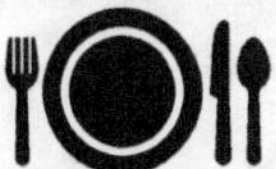 # Daily Healthy Eating Habits 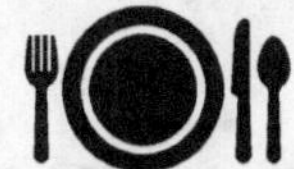

	Morning or Breakfast	Mid Day Or Lunch	Late Afternoon or Dinner	Evening Or Snacks
WATER- Drink 8-10 glasses or 3 L through out the day				
Veggies & Fruits- try to eat 5 servings each day				
Protein- Eat a palm size at each meal				
Healthy Fats- Eat fingertip - thumb size at each meal				
Follow Hand Portion Sizes at each meal				
Listen to Hunger & Fullness Cues				
Eat Mindfully & Slowly- Follow the 20 min meal				
Stop eating starchy carbs at 7pm				
Followed the 80/20 or 90/10 rule				
Any skipped meals				

Daily Exercise Plan

Activity	Length of W/O	Weight	Reps	Sets	Speed	Distance	Calories Burned

My Daily Reflections

Date:

★ Top 3 Daily Goals ★

My Action Steps To Help Me Reach My Daily Goals Are:

- [ ] _______________________
- [ ] _______________________
- [ ] _______________________

♥ My Top 3 Strengths Are ♥

Today I Found Happiness In

- [ ] _______________________
- [ ] _______________________
- [ ] _______________________

3 Things I Love About My Body

I Am Grateful For

- [ ] _______________________
- [ ] _______________________
- [ ] _______________________

Daily Meal Planner

MEAL PLAN		Macros Counts
Breakfast		Calories______ Carbs:_______ Protein:______ Fats:________
Mid Morning		Calories______ Carbs:_______ Protein:______ Fats:________
Lunch		Calories______ Carbs:_______ Protein:______ Fats:________
Afternoon		Calories______ Carbs:_______ Protein:______ Fats:________
Dinner		Calories______ Carbs:_______ Protein:______ Fats:________

	Calories	Carbs	Protein	Fats
Calculated Macros				
Daily Totals				

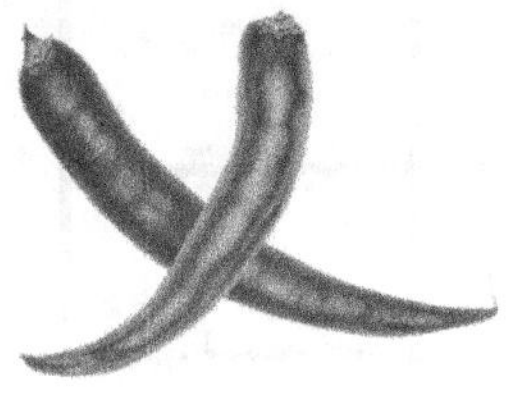
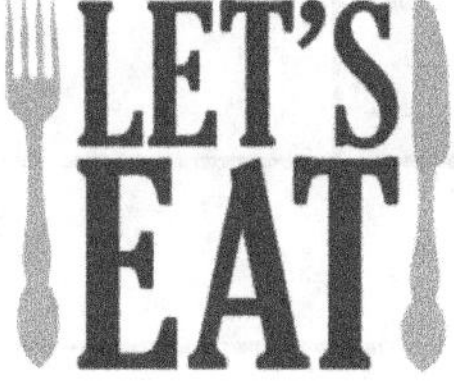

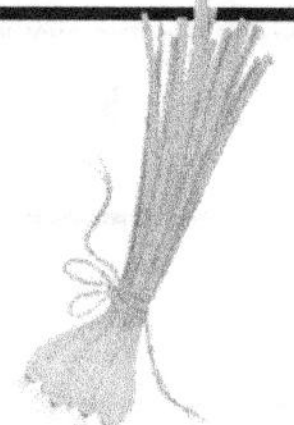

Daily Healthy Eating Habits

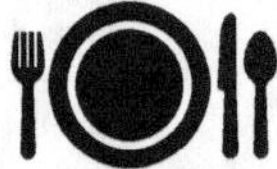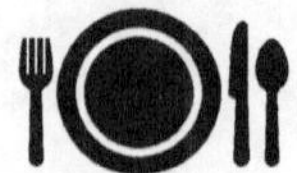

	Morning or Breakfast	Mid Day Or Lunch	Late Afternoon or Dinner	Evening Or Snacks
WATER- Drink 8-10 glasses or 3 L through out the day				
Veggies & Fruits- try to eat 5 servings each day				
Protein- Eat a palm size at each meal				
Healthy Fats- Eat fingertip - thumb size at each meal				
Follow Hand Portion Sizes at each meal				
Listen to Hunger & Fullness Cues				
Eat Mindfully & Slowly- Follow the 20 min meal				
Stop eating starchy carbs at 7pm				
Followed the 80/20 or 90/10 rule				
Any skipped meals				

Daily Exercise Plan

Activity	Length of W/O	Weight	Reps	Sets	Speed	Distance	Calories Burned

My Daily Reflections

Date:

★ Top 3 Daily Goals ★

My Action Steps To Help Me Reach My Daily Goals Are:

- ☐ ______________________________
- ☐ ______________________________
- ☐ ______________________________

♥ My Top 3 Strengths Are ♥

Today I Found Happiness In

- ☐ ______________________________
- ☐ ______________________________
- ☐ ______________________________

3 Things I Love About My Body

I Am Grateful For

- ☐ ______________________________
- ☐ ______________________________
- ☐ ______________________________

Daily Meal Planner

MEAL PLAN		Macros Counts
Breakfast		Calories______ Carbs:______ Protein:______ Fats:______
Mid Morning		Calories______ Carbs:______ Protein:______ Fats:______
Lunch		Calories______ Carbs:______ Protein:______ Fats:______
Afternoon		Calories______ Carbs:______ Protein:______ Fats:______
Dinner		Calories______ Carbs:______ Protein:______ Fats:______

	Calories	Carbs	Protein	Fats
Calculated Macros				
Daily Totals				

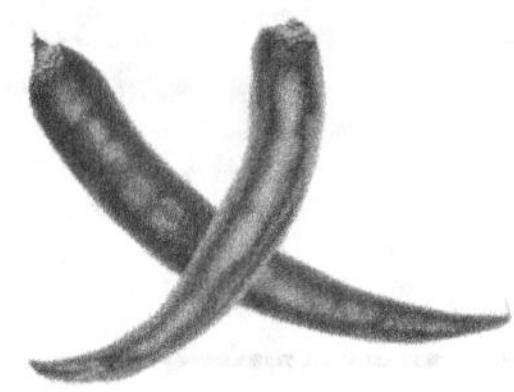
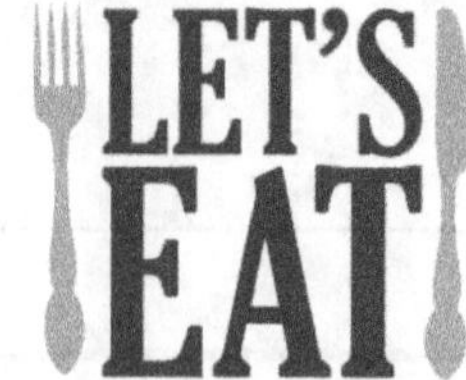

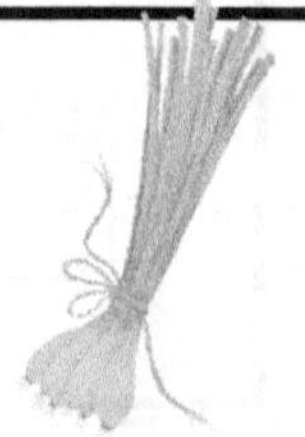

Daily Healthy Eating Habits

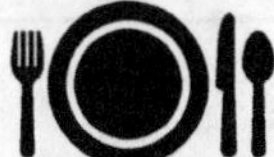 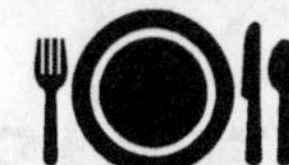

	Morning or Breakfast	Mid Day Or Lunch	Late Afternoon or Dinner	Evening Or Snacks
WATER- Drink 8-10 glasses or 3 L through out the day				
Veggies & Fruits- try to eat 5 servings each day				
Protein- Eat a palm size at each meal				
Healthy Fats- Eat fingertip - thumb size at each meal				
Follow Hand Portion Sizes at each meal				
Listen to Hunger & Fullness Cues				
Eat Mindfully & Slowly- Follow the 20 min meal				
Stop eating starchy carbs at 7pm				
Followed the 80/20 or 90/10 rule				
Any skipped meals				

Daily Exercise Plan

Activity	Length of W/O	Weight	Reps	Sets	Speed	Distance	Calories Burned

My Daily Reflections

Date:

★ Top 3 Daily Goals ★

- ☐ _______________________
- ☐ _______________________
- ☐ _______________________

My Action Steps To Help Me Reach My Daily Goals Are:

♥ My Top 3 Strengths Are ♥

- ☐ _______________________
- ☐ _______________________
- ☐ _______________________

Today I Found Happiness In

3 Things I Love About My Body

- ☐ _______________________
- ☐ _______________________
- ☐ _______________________

I Am Grateful For

Daily Meal Planner

	MEAL PLAN	Macros Counts
Breakfast		Calories______ Carbs:______ Protein:______ Fats:______
Mid Morning		Calories______ Carbs:______ Protein:______ Fats:______
Lunch		Calories______ Carbs:______ Protein:______ Fats:______
Afternoon		Calories______ Carbs:______ Protein:______ Fats:______
Dinner		Calories______ Carbs:______ Protein:______ Fats:______

	Calories	Carbs	Protein	Fats
Calculated Macros				
Daily Totals				

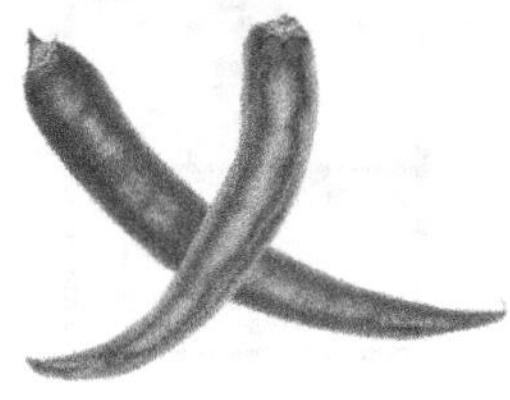

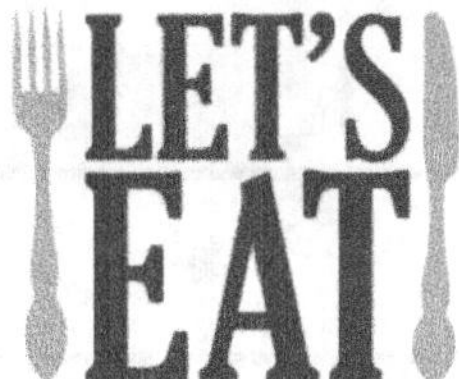

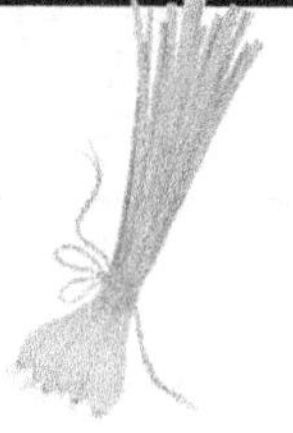

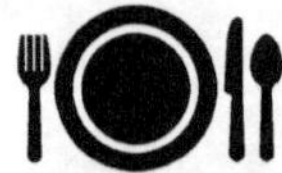 # Daily Healthy Eating Habits 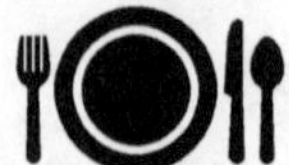

	Morning or Breakfast	Mid Day Or Lunch	Late Afternoon or Dinner	Evening Or Snacks
WATER- Drink 8-10 glasses or 3 L through out the day				
Veggies & Fruits- try to eat 5 servings each day				
Protein- Eat a palm size at each meal				
Healthy Fats- Eat fingertip - thumb size at each meal				
Follow Hand Portion Sizes at each meal				
Listen to Hunger & Fullness Cues				
Eat Mindfully & Slowly- Follow the 20 min meal				
Stop eating starchy carbs at 7pm				
Followed the 80/20 or 90/10 rule				
Any skipped meals				

Daily Exercise Plan

Activity	Length of W/O	Weight	Reps	Sets	Speed	Distance	Calories Burned

My Daily Reflections

Date:

Top 3 Daily Goals

- [ ] _______________________
- [ ] _______________________
- [ ] _______________________

My Action Steps To Help Me Reach My Daily Goals Are:

My Top 3 Strengths Are

- [ ] _______________________
- [ ] _______________________
- [ ] _______________________

Today I Found Happiness In

3 Things I Love About My Body

- [ ] _______________________
- [ ] _______________________
- [ ] _______________________

I Am Grateful For

Daily Meal Planner

MEAL PLAN		Macros Counts
Breakfast		Calories________ Carbs:________ Protein:______ Fats:__________
Mid Morning		Calories________ Carbs:________ Protein:______ Fats:__________
Lunch		Calories________ Carbs:________ Protein:______ Fats:__________
Afternoon		Calories________ Carbs:________ Protein:______ Fats:__________
Dinner		Calories________ Carbs:________ Protein:______ Fats:__________

	Calories	Carbs	Protein	Fats
Calculated Macros				
Daily Totals				

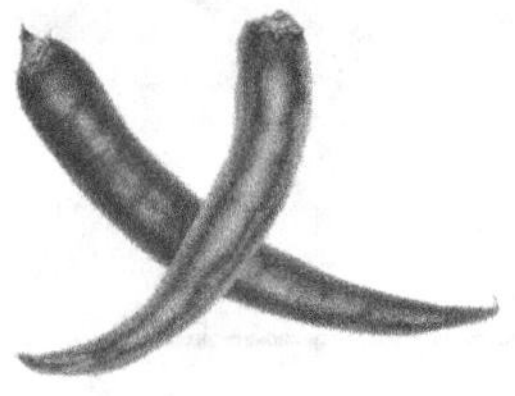

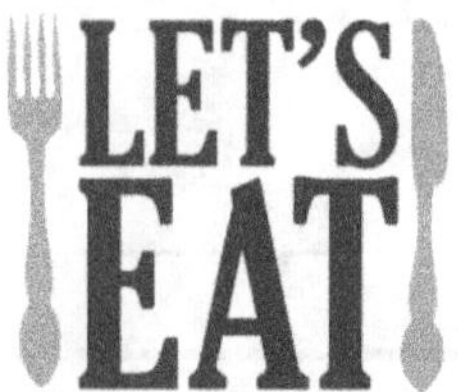

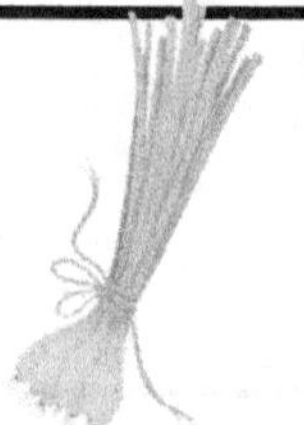

Daily Healthy Eating Habits

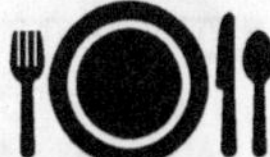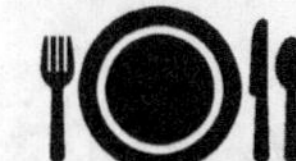

	Morning or Breakfast	Mid Day Or Lunch	Late Afternoon or Dinner	Evening Or Snacks
WATER- Drink 8-10 glasses or 3 L through out the day				
Veggies & Fruits- try to eat 5 servings each day				
Protein- Eat a palm size at each meal				
Healthy Fats- Eat fingertip - thumb size at each meal				
Follow Hand Portion Sizes at each meal				
Listen to Hunger & Fullness Cues				
Eat Mindfully & Slowly- Follow the 20 min meal				
Stop eating starchy carbs at 7pm				
Followed the 80/20 or 90/10 rule				
Any skipped meals				

Daily Exercise Plan

Activity	Length of W/O	Weight	Reps	Sets	Speed	Distance	Calories Burned

My Daily Reflections

Date:

★ Top 3 Daily Goals ★

My Action Steps To Help Me
Reach My Daily Goals Are:

- ☐ _______________________
- ☐ _______________________
- ☐ _______________________

♥ My Top 3 Strengths Are ♥

Today I Found Happiness In

- ☐ _______________________
- ☐ _______________________
- ☐ _______________________

3 Things I Love About My Body

I Am Grateful For

- ☐ _______________________
- ☐ _______________________
- ☐ _______________________

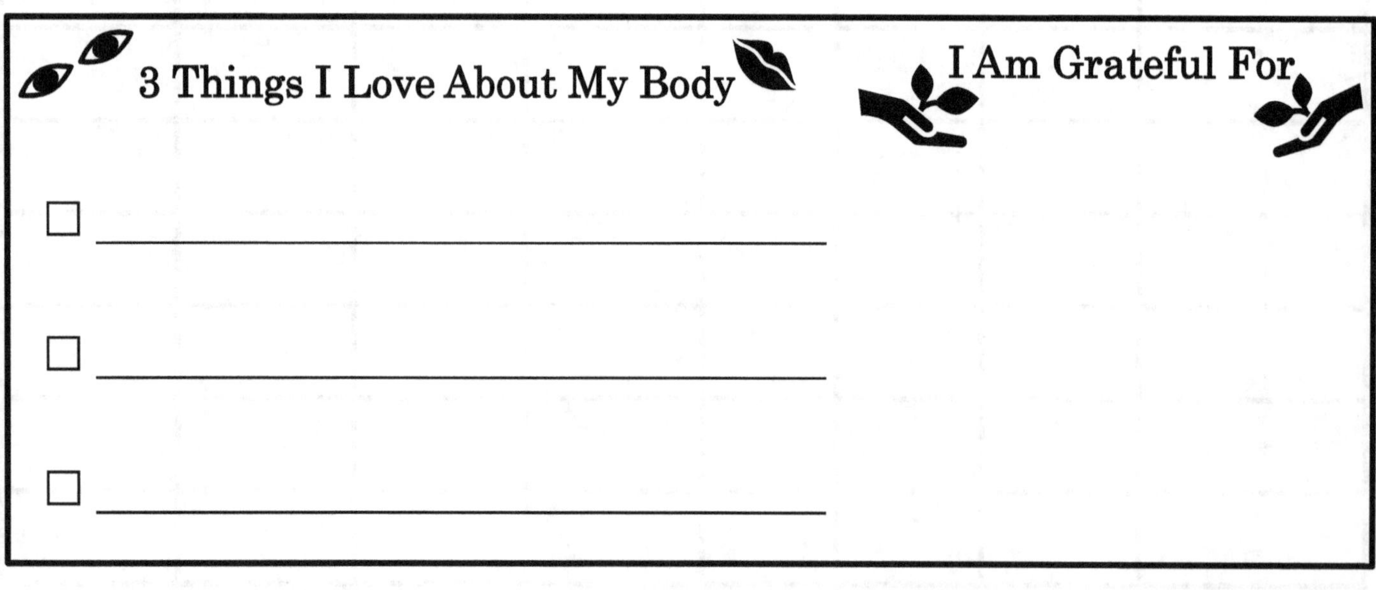

Daily Meal Planner

	MEAL PLAN	Macros Counts
Breakfast		Calories_______ Carbs:_______ Protein:_______ Fats:_______
Mid Morning		Calories_______ Carbs:_______ Protein:_______ Fats:_______
Lunch		Calories_______ Carbs:_______ Protein:_______ Fats:_______
Afternoon		Calories_______ Carbs:_______ Protein:_______ Fats:_______
Dinner		Calories_______ Carbs:_______ Protein:_______ Fats:_______

	Calories	Carbs	Protein	Fats
Calculated Macros				
Daily Totals				

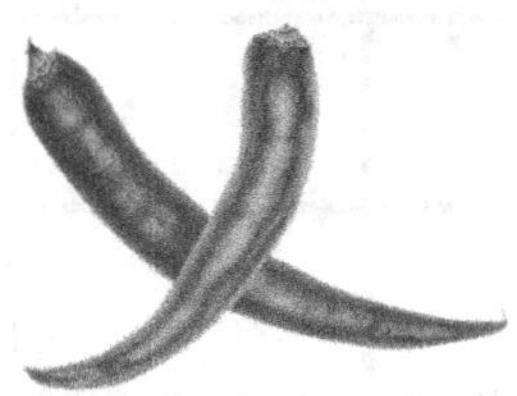
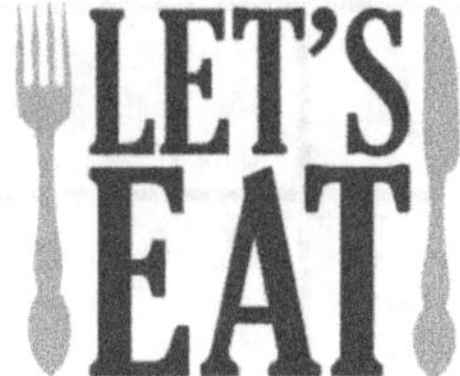

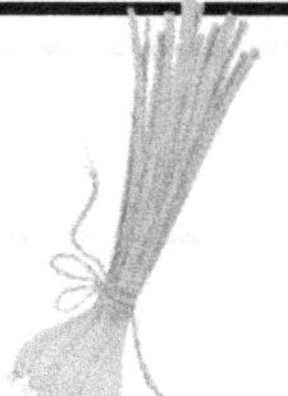

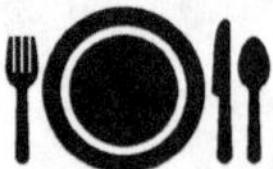 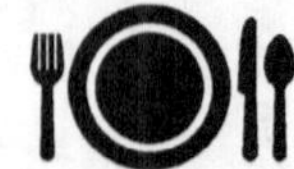

Daily Healthy Eating Habits

	Morning or Breakfast	Mid Day Or Lunch	Late Afternoon or Dinner	Evening Or Snacks
WATER- Drink 8-10 glasses or 3 L through out the day				
Veggies & Fruits- try to eat 5 servings each day				
Protein- Eat a palm size at each meal				
Healthy Fats- Eat fingertip - thumb size at each meal				
Follow Hand Portion Sizes at each meal				
Listen to Hunger & Fullness Cues				
Eat Mindfully & Slowly- Follow the 20 min meal				
Stop eating starchy carbs at 7pm				
Followed the 80/20 or 90/10 rule				
Any skipped meals				

Daily Exercise Plan

Activity	Length of W/O	Weight	Reps	Sets	Speed	Distance	Calories Burned

<table>
<tr><td>Week Of:</td><td>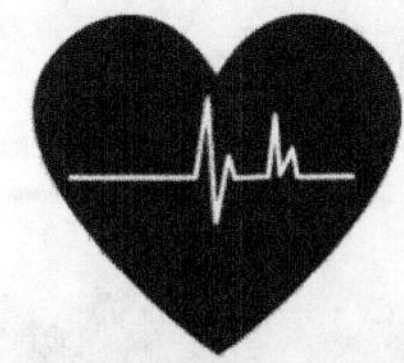</td><td colspan="2">Track Your Blood Sugar</td></tr>
</table>

Date	Wake Up	Pre-Lunch	Afternoon	Pre-Dinner	Bedtime

Results					
High					
Good					
Low					

Note Any Changes

WEEK 4 FROM: _______________

100 Low Carb Swaps Cheat Sheet

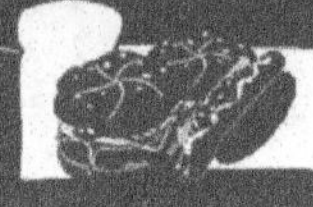
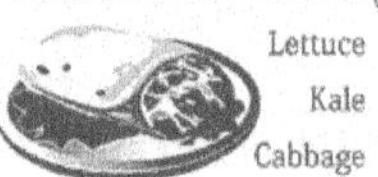
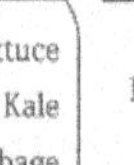
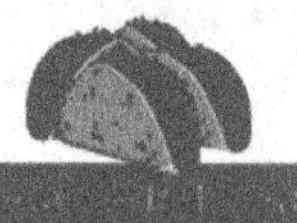
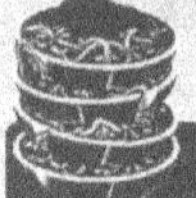

Kale leaves
Lettuce leaves
Thick sliced cucumbers
Roasted Portobello
mushroom caps
Napa or Chinese cabbage

Save minimum 18 grams of carbs per 2 slices of bread and 21 grams for each bun

Lettuce
Kale
Cabbage

Save 32 to 43 grams of carbs in traditional wraps and tortillas

Flax Crackers
Parmesan cheese crisps

Almond flour or coconut flour crackers (recipes online)

Cucumbers, raw zucchini, celery and carrots

Save 6 or more grams of carbs per 5 crackers

Put all the fillings on leaves of lettuce, kale or cabbage

Save 23 grams of carbs in taco size tortillas

Sliced nuts
Real bacon bits
Parmesan cheese crisps
Crumbled flax crackers
Sunflower seeds

Save 15 grams of carbs per ounce

Spiral cut zucchini
Japanese shirataki noodles
Spaghetti squash
Kelp noodles

Save 37.3 grams of carbs for each 1 cup of pasta

Zucchini slices
Eggplant slices

Save 21 grams of carbs by replacing just 2 noodles

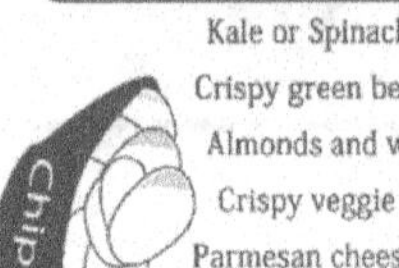
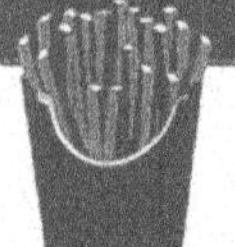

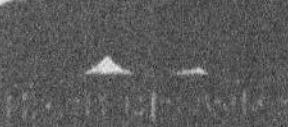
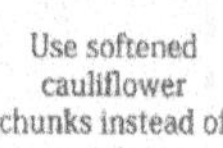

Kale or Spinach chips
Crispy green bean fries
Almonds and walnuts
Crispy veggie sticks
Parmesan cheese crisps
Pepperoni chips
Pickles
Almond flour or coconut flour crackers (recipes online)
Flax crackers Roasted seasoned seaweed

Save an average of 114 grams of carbs that are in 8 ounces of chips

Baked carrot sticks
Crispy green bean fries
Crispy turnip fries
Crispy daikon Fries
Crispy zucchini Fries

(recipes are online for all above swaps)

Save a minimum of 56 grams of carbs in a 1-cup serving

Mashed cauliflower Flavor with a little cheese, garlic, butter, or sour cream

Save 18 grams of carbs per ½ cup

Use spaghetti squash or cauliflower instead of potatoes, fry up as usual

Save 18 grams of carbs per ½ cup

Use softened cauliflower chunks instead of potatoes

Save 20 grams of carbs with each 1-cup serving

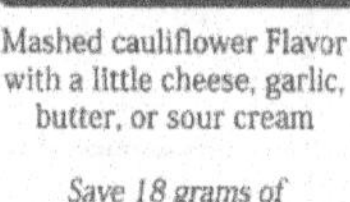

Portobello mushroom cap

Cauliflower Pizza Crust (recipes online)

Coconut flour pizza crust (recipes online)

Save a minimum of 16 grams per 2 slices of crust

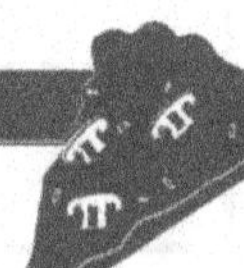

Eggs any style
Bacon/Sausage and eggs
Breakfast sandwiches wrapped in a firm omelet instead of English muffin, bagels or breads
Eggs with salsa and flax cracker with cream cheese
Bacon, onion and tomato lettuce wraps
Omelets with veggies, meats, cheese
Egg bakes and skillets with meats, veggies
Pancakes and waffles made with coconut or almond flour
Smoked salmon with cream cheese, tomatoes and onions
Smoked salmon scrambled eggs with chives/sour cream
Flax crackers and cheese
Green smoothie
Deviled eggs
Deviled eggs with a shrimp and avocado on top
Hard-boiled eggs cut in half with guacamole/bacon on top
Flax crackers with peanut or almond butter and a few mashed berries or sugar free jam on top
Flourless egg and cottage cheese muffins (recipe online)
Egg frittatas
Cream cheese pancakes (recipe online)

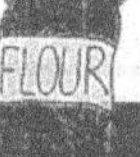
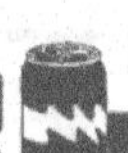
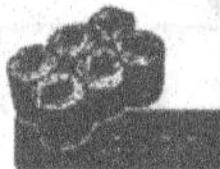

Blueberries, raspberries, or strawberries with heavy whipping cream
Sugar free Jell-O™ with heavy whipping cream
Milk shake with almond milk, cocoa powder, and nut butter
Sour cream with stevia and berries
Strawberry with almond or peanut butter
Atkins™ bars and shakes
Coconut-cashew chocolate truffles (recipe online)
Almond flour cookies and muffins (recipes online)
Chocolate and flan layered mini cakes (recipe online)
Strawberries dipped in sugar free chocolate
Strawberries dipped in sugar free caramel
Sugar free ice pops

Almond Flour
Coconut flour

Crushed nut crusting
Save about 40 grams of carbs in ½ cup of white flour

Zero calorie flavored seltzers

Save 39 grams of pure sugar carbs in a 12-ounce serving

Sashimi

Sushi cut and hand rolls without rice

Save 26 or more grams of carbs in each roll

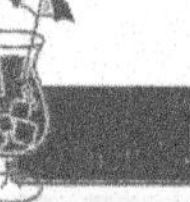
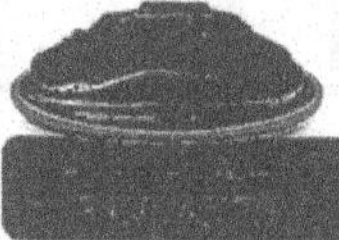
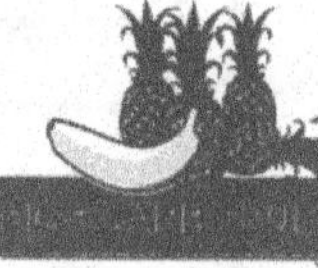
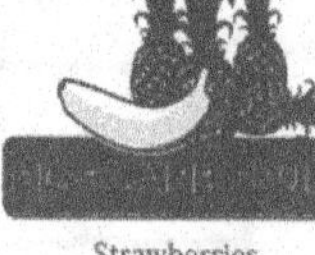

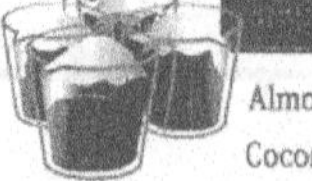

Straight spirits (vodka, gin, whiskey) mixed with club soda or diet tonic

Wine

Save a minimum of 15 grams of carbs per drink

Almond flour pancakes (recipes online)

Save 20 grams of carbs in just 2 buttermilk pancakes

Strawberries
Blueberries
Raspberries
Cantaloupe

Save 15 plus grams per fruit

Almond flour
Coconut flour

Save 23 grams of carbs per half cup

My Daily Reflections

Date:

Top 3 Daily Goals

- ☐ _______________
- ☐ _______________
- ☐ _______________

My Action Steps To Help Me Reach My Daily Goals Are:

My Top 3 Strengths Are

- ☐ _______________
- ☐ _______________
- ☐ _______________

Today I Found Happiness In

3 Things I Love About My Body

- ☐ _______________
- ☐ _______________
- ☐ _______________

I Am Grateful For

Daily Meal Planner

	MEAL PLAN	Macros Counts
Breakfast		Calories______ Carbs:______ Protein:______ Fats:______
Mid Morning		Calories______ Carbs:______ Protein:______ Fats:______
Lunch		Calories______ Carbs:______ Protein:______ Fats:______
Afternoon		Calories______ Carbs:______ Protein:______ Fats:______
Dinner		Calories______ Carbs:______ Protein:______ Fats:______

	Calories	Carbs	Protein	Fats
Calculated Macros				
Daily Totals				

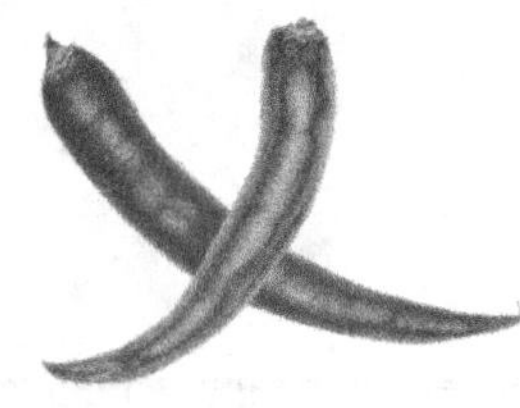
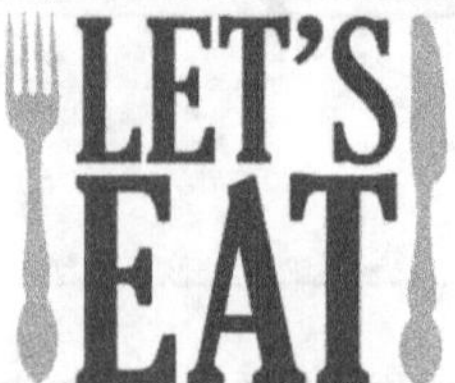

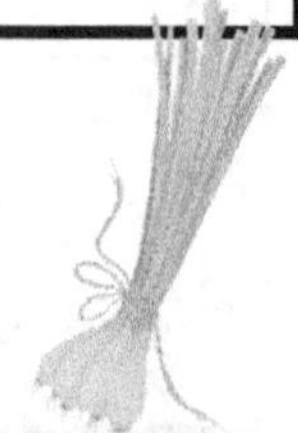

Daily Healthy Eating Habits

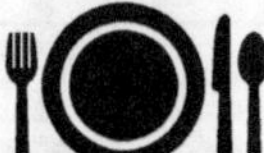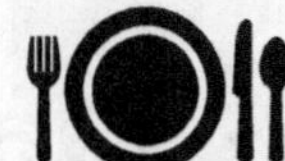

	Morning or Breakfast	Mid Day Or Lunch	Late Afternoon or Dinner	Evening Or Snacks
WATER- Drink 8-10 glasses or 3 L through out the day				
Veggies & Fruits- try to eat 5 servings each day				
Protein- Eat a palm size at each meal				
Healthy Fats- Eat fingertip - thumb size at each meal				
Follow Hand Portion Sizes at each meal				
Listen to Hunger & Fullness Cues				
Eat Mindfully & Slowly- Follow the 20 min meal				
Stop eating starchy carbs at 7pm				
Followed the 80/20 or 90/10 rule				
Any skipped meals				

Daily Exercise Plan

Activity	Length of W/O	Weight	Reps	Sets	Speed	Distance	Calories Burned

My Daily Reflections

Date:

★ Top 3 Daily Goals ★

My Action Steps To Help Me Reach My Daily Goals Are:

- ☐ _______________________
- ☐ _______________________
- ☐ _______________________

♥ My Top 3 Strengths Are ♥

Today I Found Happiness In

- ☐ _______________________
- ☐ _______________________
- ☐ _______________________

3 Things I Love About My Body

I Am Grateful For

- ☐ _______________________
- ☐ _______________________
- ☐ _______________________

Daily Meal Planner

MEAL PLAN		Macros Counts
Breakfast		Calories________ Carbs:________ Protein:______ Fats:__________
Mid Morning		Calories________ Carbs:________ Protein:______ Fats:__________
Lunch		Calories________ Carbs:________ Protein:______ Fats:__________
Afternoon		Calories________ Carbs:________ Protein:______ Fats:__________
Dinner		Calories________ Carbs:________ Protein:______ Fats:__________

	Calories	Carbs	Protein	Fats
Calculated Macros				
Daily Totals				

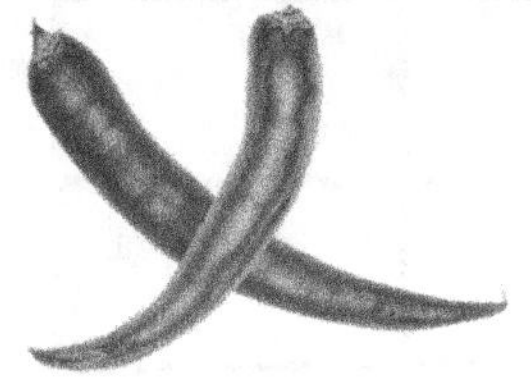
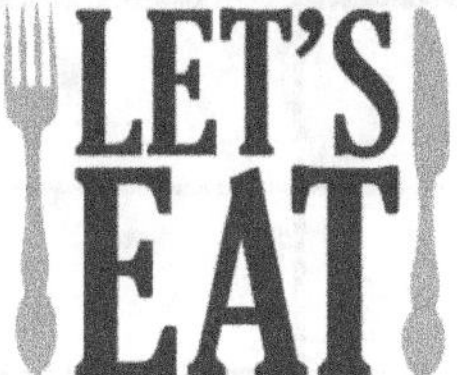

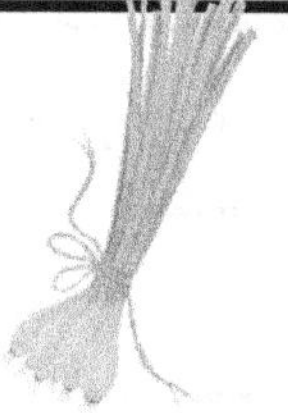

Daily Healthy Eating Habits

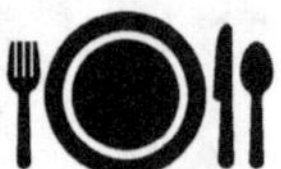 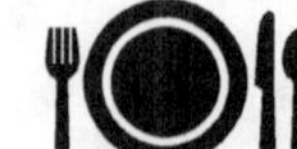

	Morning or Breakfast	Mid Day Or Lunch	Late Afternoon or Dinner	Evening Or Snacks
WATER- Drink 8-10 glasses or 3 L through out the day				
Veggies & Fruits- try to eat 5 servings each day				
Protein- Eat a palm size at each meal				
Healthy Fats- Eat fingertip - thumb size at each meal				
Follow Hand Portion Sizes at each meal				
Listen to Hunger & Fullness Cues				
Eat Mindfully & Slowly- Follow the 20 min meal				
Stop eating starchy carbs at 7pm				
Followed the 80/20 or 90/10 rule				
Any skipped meals				

Daily Exercise Plan

Activity	Length of W/O	Weight	Reps	Sets	Speed	Distance	Calories Burned

My Daily Reflections

Date:

✦✦ Top 3 Daily Goals ✦✦

☐ _______________________________

☐ _______________________________

☐ _______________________________

My Action Steps To Help Me Reach My Daily Goals Are:

♥ My Top 3 Strengths Are ♥

☐ _______________________________

☐ _______________________________

☐ _______________________________

Today I Found Happiness In

3 Things I Love About My Body

☐ _______________________________

☐ _______________________________

☐ _______________________________

I Am Grateful For

Daily Meal Planner

MEAL PLAN		Macros Counts
Breakfast		Calories_______ Carbs:_______ Protein:_______ Fats:_________
Mid Morning		Calories_______ Carbs:_______ Protein:_______ Fats:_________
Lunch		Calories_______ Carbs:_______ Protein:_______ Fats:_________
Afternoon		Calories_______ Carbs:_______ Protein:_______ Fats:_________
Dinner		Calories_______ Carbs:_______ Protein:_______ Fats:_________

	Calories	Carbs	Protein	Fats
Calculated Macros				
Daily Totals				

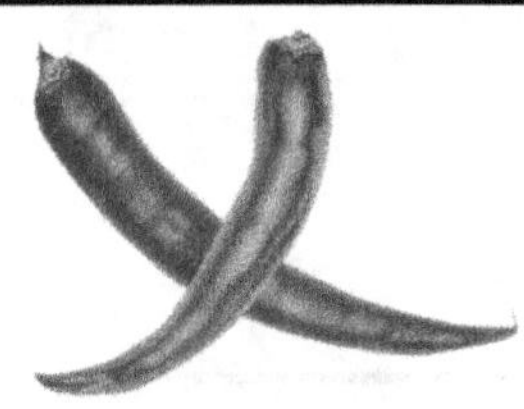
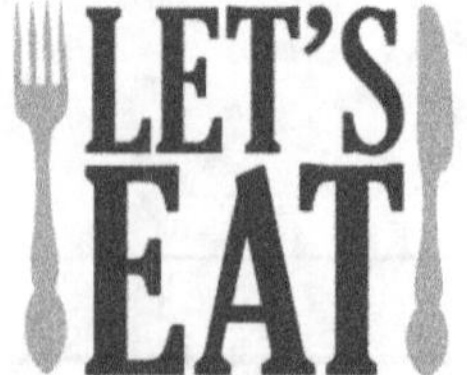

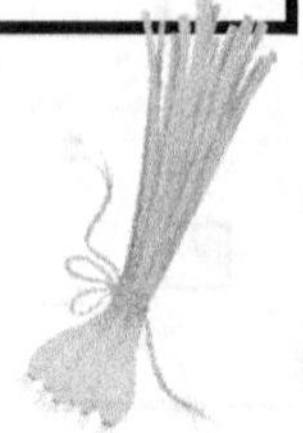

 # Daily Healthy Eating Habits 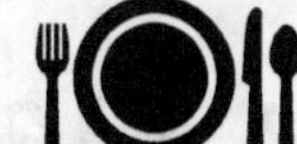

	Morning or Breakfast	Mid Day Or Lunch	Late Afternoon or Dinner	Evening Or Snacks
WATER- Drink 8-10 glasses or 3 L through out the day				
Veggies & Fruits- try to eat 5 servings each day				
Protein- Eat a palm size at each meal				
Healthy Fats- Eat fingertip - thumb size at each meal				
Follow Hand Portion Sizes at each meal				
Listen to Hunger & Fullness Cues				
Eat Mindfully & Slowly- Follow the 20 min meal				
Stop eating starchy carbs at 7pm				
Followed the 80/20 or 90/10 rule				
Any skipped meals				

Daily Exercise Plan

Activity	Length of W/O	Weight	Reps	Sets	Speed	Distance	Calories Burned

My Daily Reflections

Date:

Top 3 Daily Goals

My Action Steps To Help Me
Reach My Daily Goals Are:

- [ ] _______________________
- [ ] _______________________
- [ ] _______________________

My Top 3 Strengths Are

Today I Found Happiness In

- [ ] _______________________
- [ ] _______________________
- [ ] _______________________

3 Things I Love About My Body

I Am Grateful For

- [ ] _______________________
- [ ] _______________________
- [ ] _______________________

Daily Meal Planner

MEAL PLAN		Macros Counts
Breakfast		Calories______ Carbs:_______ Protein:______ Fats:________
Mid Morning		Calories______ Carbs:_______ Protein:______ Fats:________
Lunch		Calories______ Carbs:_______ Protein:______ Fats:________
Afternoon		Calories______ Carbs:_______ Protein:______ Fats:________
Dinner		Calories______ Carbs:_______ Protein:______ Fats:________

	Calories	Carbs	Protein	Fats
Calculated Macros				
Daily Totals				

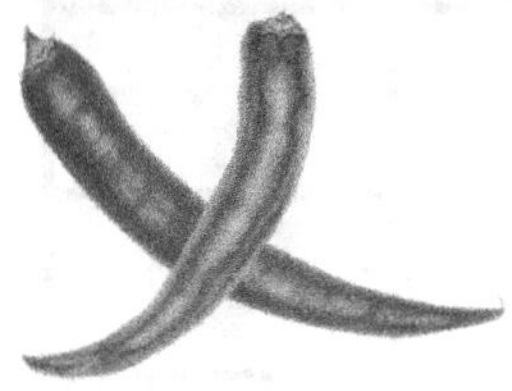

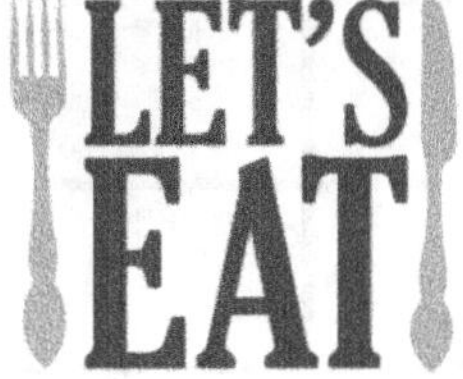

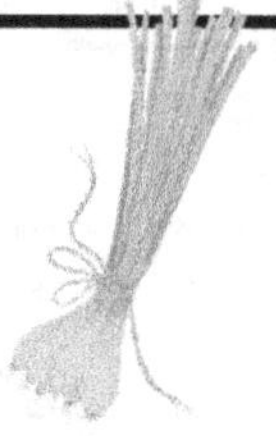

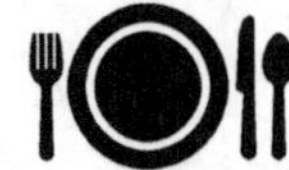 Daily Healthy Eating Habits 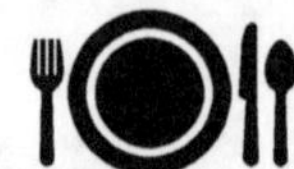

	Morning or Breakfast	Mid Day Or Lunch	Late Afternoon or Dinner	Evening Or Snacks
WATER- Drink 8-10 glasses or 3 L through out the day				
Veggies & Fruits- try to eat 5 servings each day				
Protein- Eat a palm size at each meal				
Healthy Fats- Eat fingertip - thumb size at each meal				
Follow Hand Portion Sizes at each meal				
Listen to Hunger & Fullness Cues				
Eat Mindfully & Slowly- Follow the 20 min meal				
Stop eating starchy carbs at 7pm				
Followed the 80/20 or 90/10 rule				
Any skipped meals				

Daily Exercise Plan

Activity	Length of W/O	Weight	Reps	Sets	Speed	Distance	Calories Burned

My Daily Reflections

Date:

★ Top 3 Daily Goals ★

My Action Steps To Help Me
Reach My Daily Goals Are:

- [ ] _______________________
- [ ] _______________________
- [ ] _______________________

♥ My Top 3 Strengths Are ♥

Today I Found Happiness In

- [ ] _______________________
- [ ] _______________________
- [ ] _______________________

3 Things I Love About My Body

I Am Grateful For

- [ ] _______________________
- [ ] _______________________
- [ ] _______________________

Daily Meal Planner

MEAL PLAN		Macros Counts
Breakfast		Calories________ Carbs:________ Protein:________ Fats:__________
Mid Morning		Calories________ Carbs:________ Protein:________ Fats:__________
Lunch		Calories________ Carbs:________ Protein:________ Fats:__________
Afternoon		Calories________ Carbs:________ Protein:________ Fats:__________
Dinner		Calories________ Carbs:________ Protein:________ Fats:__________

	Calories	Carbs	Protein	Fats
Calculated Macros				
Daily Totals				

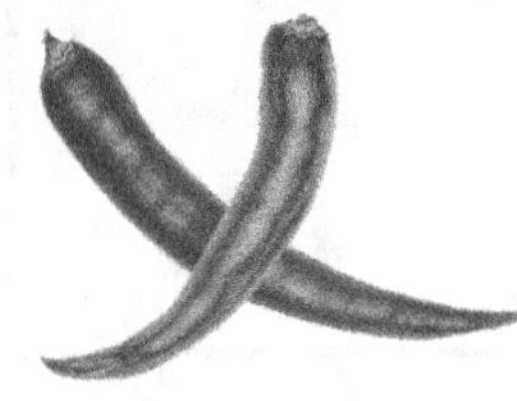

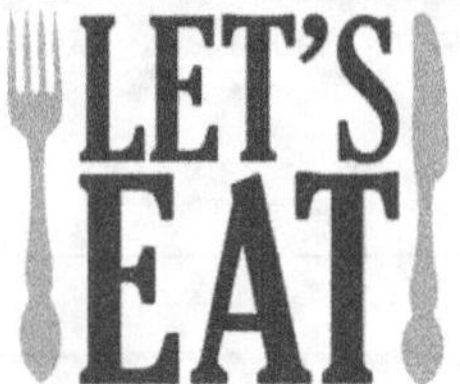

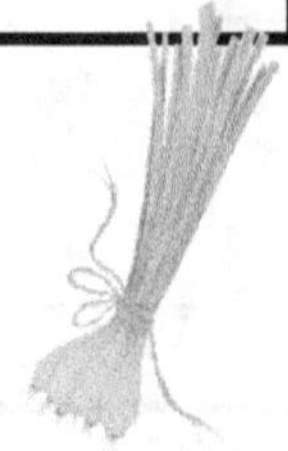

Daily Healthy Eating Habits

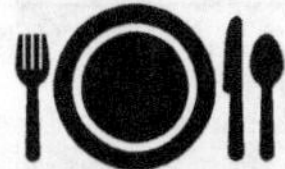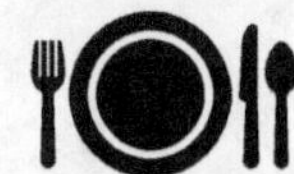

	Morning or Breakfast	Mid Day Or Lunch	Late Afternoon or Dinner	Evening Or Snacks
WATER- Drink 8-10 glasses or 3 L through out the day				
Veggies & Fruits- try to eat 5 servings each day				
Protein- Eat a palm size at each meal				
Healthy Fats- Eat fingertip - thumb size at each meal				
Follow Hand Portion Sizes at each meal				
Listen to Hunger & Fullness Cues				
Eat Mindfully & Slowly- Follow the 20 min meal				
Stop eating starchy carbs at 7pm				
Followed the 80/20 or 90/10 rule				
Any skipped meals				

Daily Exercise Plan

Activity	Length of W/O	Weight	Reps	Sets	Speed	Distance	Calories Burned

My Daily Reflections

Date:

★ Top 3 Daily Goals ★

- [ ] _______________________________
- [ ] _______________________________
- [ ] _______________________________

My Action Steps To Help Me Reach My Daily Goals Are:

♥ My Top 3 Strengths Are ♥

- [ ] _______________________________
- [ ] _______________________________
- [ ] _______________________________

Today I Found Happiness In

3 Things I Love About My Body

- [ ] _______________________________
- [ ] _______________________________
- [ ] _______________________________

I Am Grateful For

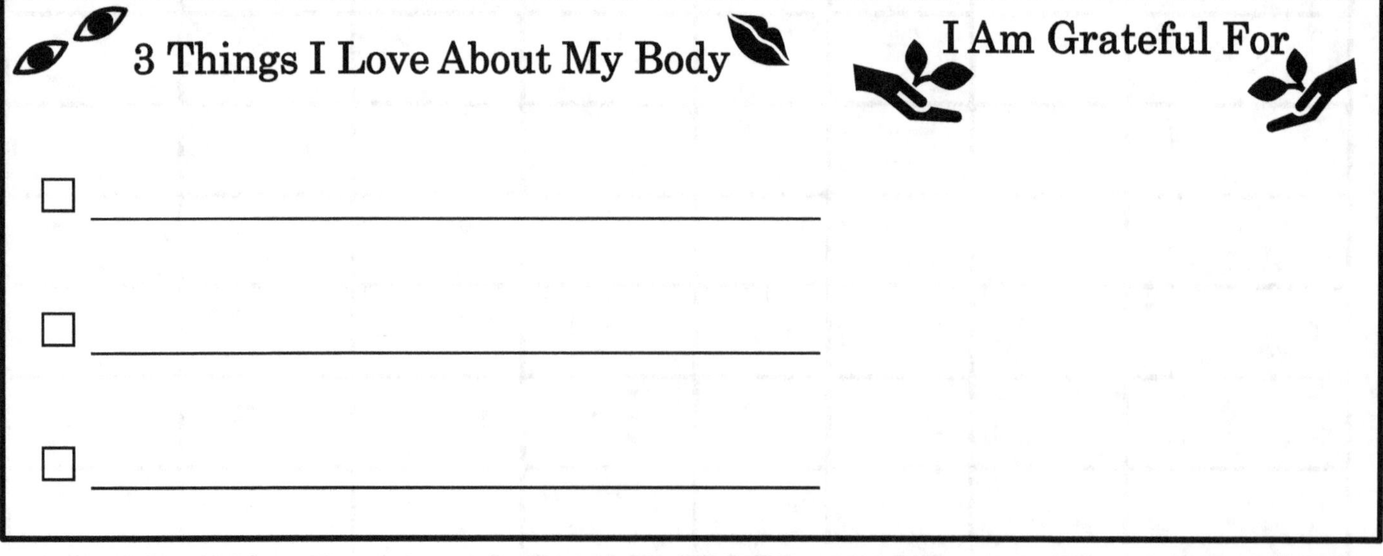

Daily Meal Planner

MEAL PLAN		Macros Counts
Breakfast		Calories________ Carbs:________ Protein:________ Fats:________
Mid Morning		Calories________ Carbs:________ Protein:________ Fats:________
Lunch		Calories________ Carbs:________ Protein:________ Fats:________
Afternoon		Calories________ Carbs:________ Protein:________ Fats:________
Dinner		Calories________ Carbs:________ Protein:________ Fats:________

	Calories	Carbs	Protein	Fats
Calculated Macros				
Daily Totals				

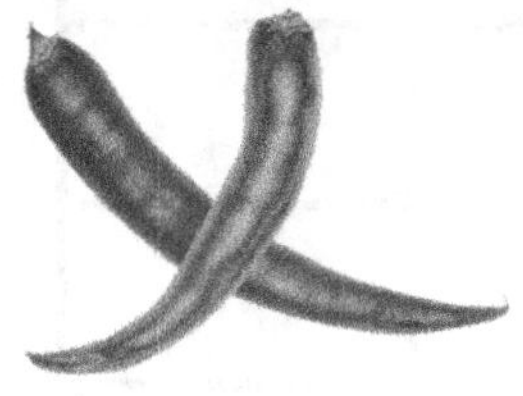

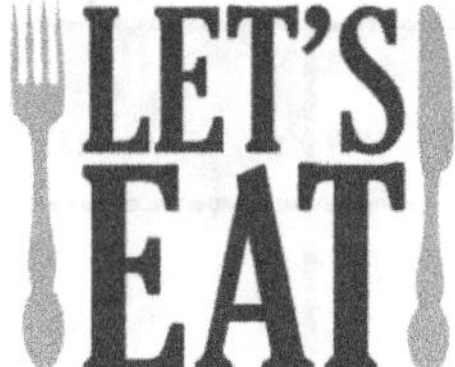

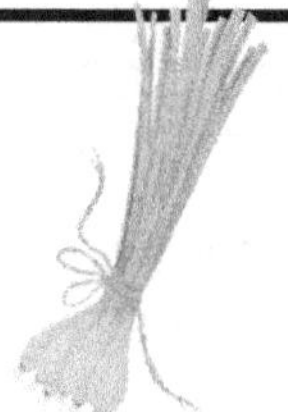

Daily Healthy Eating Habits

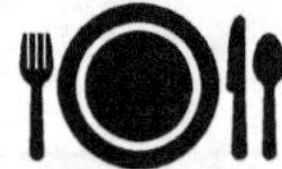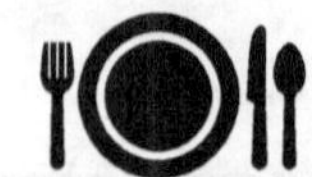

	Morning or Breakfast	Mid Day Or Lunch	Late Afternoon or Dinner	Evening Or Snacks
WATER- Drink 8-10 glasses or 3 L through out the day				
Veggies & Fruits- try to eat 5 servings each day				
Protein- Eat a palm size at each meal				
Healthy Fats- Eat fingertip - thumb size at each meal				
Follow Hand Portion Sizes at each meal				
Listen to Hunger & Fullness Cues				
Eat Mindfully & Slowly- Follow the 20 min meal				
Stop eating starchy carbs at 7pm				
Followed the 80/20 or 90/10 rule				
Any skipped meals				

Daily Exercise Plan

Activity	Length of W/O	Weight	Reps	Sets	Speed	Distance	Calories Burned

My Daily Reflections

Date:

Top 3 Daily Goals

- ☐ _______________________
- ☐ _______________________
- ☐ _______________________

My Action Steps To Help Me Reach My Daily Goals Are:

My Top 3 Strengths Are

- ☐ _______________________
- ☐ _______________________
- ☐ _______________________

Today I Found Happiness In

3 Things I Love About My Body

I Am Grateful For

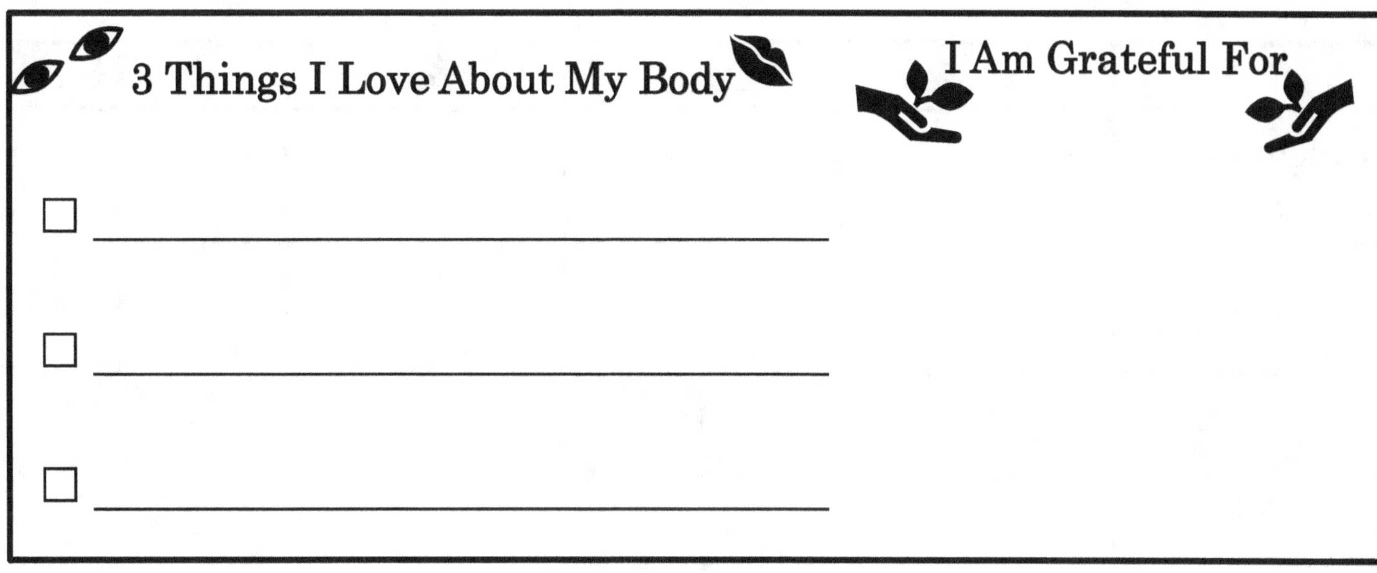

- ☐ _______________________
- ☐ _______________________
- ☐ _______________________

Daily Meal Planner

MEAL PLAN		Macros Counts
Breakfast		Calories_______ Carbs:_______ Protein:_______ Fats:_________
Mid Morning		Calories_______ Carbs:_______ Protein:_______ Fats:_________
Lunch		Calories_______ Carbs:_______ Protein:_______ Fats:_________
Afternoon		Calories_______ Carbs:_______ Protein:_______ Fats:_________
Dinner		Calories_______ Carbs:_______ Protein:_______ Fats:_________

	Calories	Carbs	Protein	Fats
Calculated Macros				
Daily Totals				

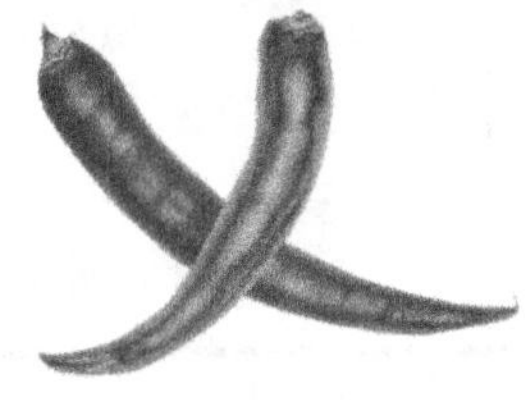
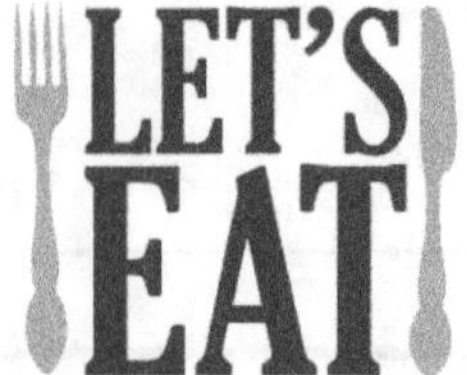

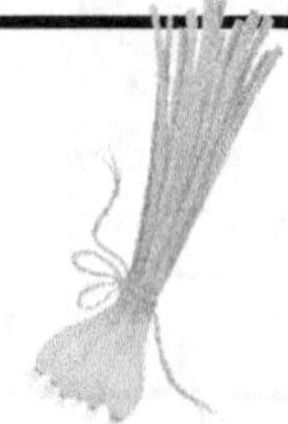

Daily Healthy Eating Habits

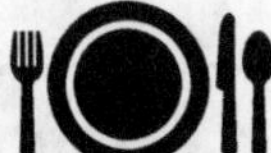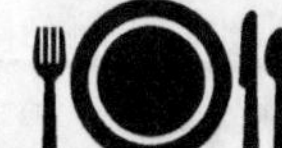

	Morning or Breakfast	Mid Day Or Lunch	Late Afternoon or Dinner	Evening Or Snacks
WATER- Drink 8-10 glasses or 3 L through out the day	⬭ ⬭ ⬭ ⬭ ⬭ ⬭ ⬭ ⬭			
Veggies & Fruits- try to eat 5 servings each day	🍎 🍎 🍎 🍎 🍎 🍎 🍎			
Protein- Eat a palm size at each meal				
Healthy Fats- Eat fingertip - thumb size at each meal				
Follow Hand Portion Sizes at each meal				
Listen to Hunger & Fullness Cues				
Eat Mindfully & Slowly- Follow the 20 min meal				
Stop eating starchy carbs at 7pm				
Followed the 80/20 or 90/10 rule				
Any skipped meals				

Daily Exercise Plan

Activity	Length of W/O	Weight	Reps	Sets	Speed	Distance	Calories Burned

<table>
<tr><td>Week Of:</td><td>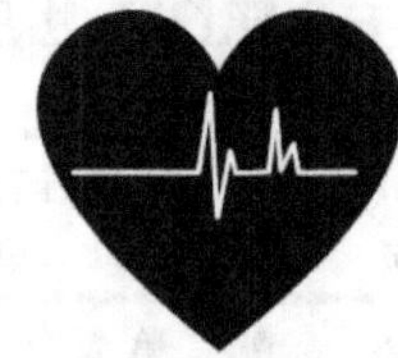</td><td>Track Your Blood Sugar</td></tr>
</table>

Date	Wake Up	Pre-Lunch	Afternoon	Pre-Dinner	Bedtime

Results

High				
Good				
Low				

Note Any Changes

WEEK 5 FROM: _______________

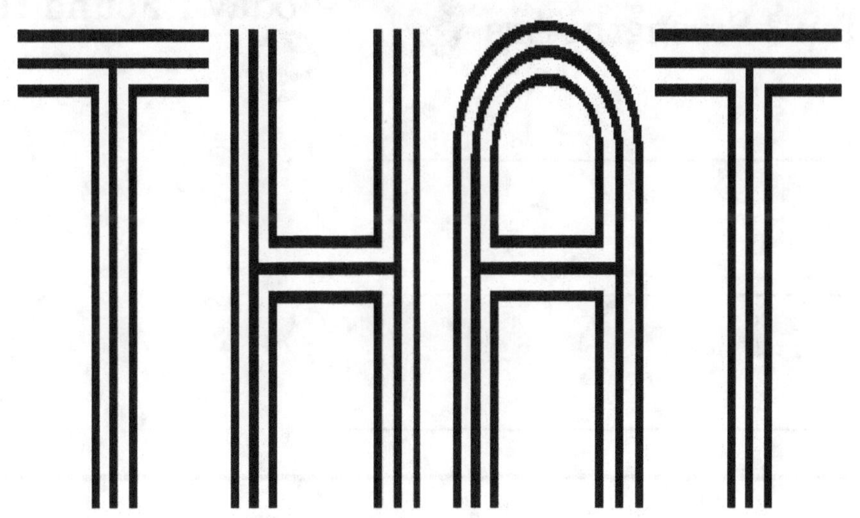

CREATE
HABITS
THAT
COMPLEMENT
YOUR GOALS

My Daily Reflections

Date:

⭐ Top 3 Daily Goals ⭐

- ☐ ___________________________
- ☐ ___________________________
- ☐ ___________________________

My Action Steps To Help Me Reach My Daily Goals Are:

♥ My Top 3 Strengths Are ♥

- ☐ ___________________________
- ☐ ___________________________
- ☐ ___________________________

Today I Found Happiness In

3 Things I Love About My Body

- ☐ ___________________________
- ☐ ___________________________
- ☐ ___________________________

I Am Grateful For

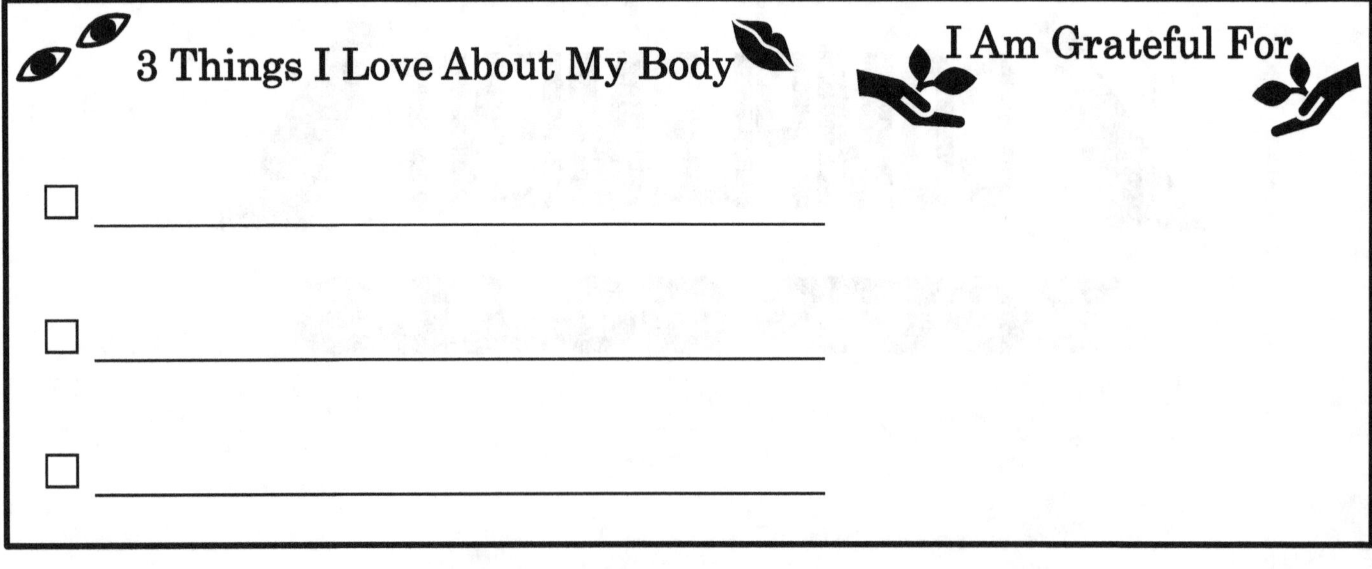

Daily Meal Planner

MEAL PLAN		Macros Counts
Breakfast		Calories________ Carbs:_________ Protein:_______ Fats:__________
Mid Morning		Calories________ Carbs:_________ Protein:_______ Fats:__________
Lunch		Calories________ Carbs:_________ Protein:_______ Fats:__________
Afternoon		Calories________ Carbs:_________ Protein:_______ Fats:__________
Dinner		Calories________ Carbs:_________ Protein:_______ Fats:__________

	Calories	Carbs	Protein	Fats
Calculated Macros				
Daily Totals				

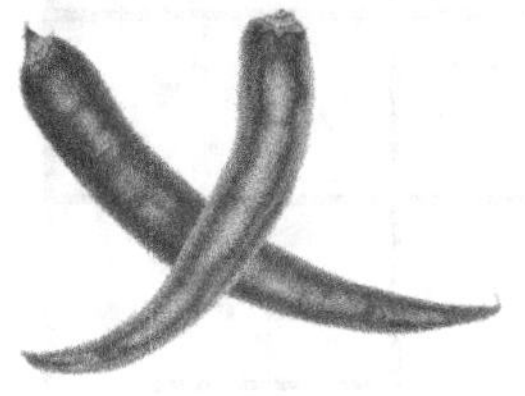
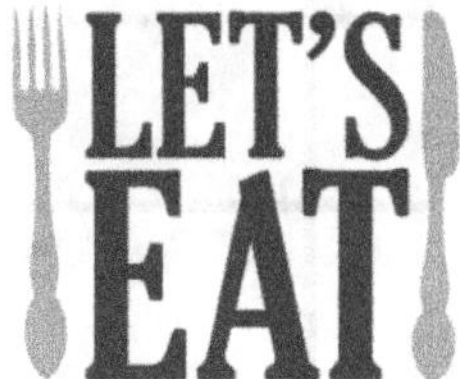

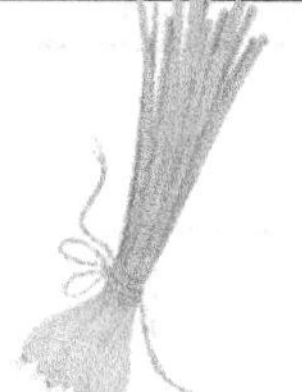

Daily Healthy Eating Habits

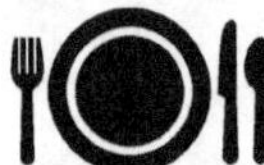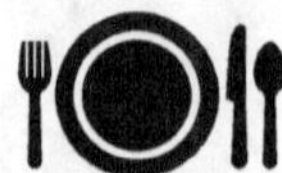

	Morning or Breakfast	Mid Day Or Lunch	Late Afternoon or Dinner	Evening Or Snacks
WATER- Drink 8-10 glasses or 3 L through out the day				
Veggies & Fruits- try to eat 5 servings each day				
Protein- Eat a palm size at each meal				
Healthy Fats- Eat fingertip - thumb size at each meal				
Follow Hand Portion Sizes at each meal				
Listen to Hunger & Fullness Cues				
Eat Mindfully & Slowly- Follow the 20 min meal				
Stop eating starchy carbs at 7pm				
Followed the 80/20 or 90/10 rule				
Any skipped meals				

Daily Exercise Plan

Activity	Length of W/O	Weight	Reps	Sets	Speed	Distance	Calories Burned

My Daily Reflections

Date:

Top 3 Daily Goals

- ☐ ________________
- ☐ ________________
- ☐ ________________

My Action Steps To Help Me Reach My Daily Goals Are:

My Top 3 Strengths Are

- ☐ ________________
- ☐ ________________
- ☐ ________________

Today I Found Happiness In

3 Things I Love About My Body

- ☐ ________________
- ☐ ________________
- ☐ ________________

I Am Grateful For

Daily Meal Planner

MEAL PLAN		Macros Counts
Breakfast		Calories_______ Carbs:_______ Protein:_______ Fats:_________
Mid Morning		Calories_______ Carbs:_______ Protein:_______ Fats:_________
Lunch		Calories_______ Carbs:_______ Protein:_______ Fats:_________
Afternoon		Calories_______ Carbs:_______ Protein:_______ Fats:_________
Dinner		Calories_______ Carbs:_______ Protein:_______ Fats:_________

	Calories	Carbs	Protein	Fats
Calculated Macros				
Daily Totals				

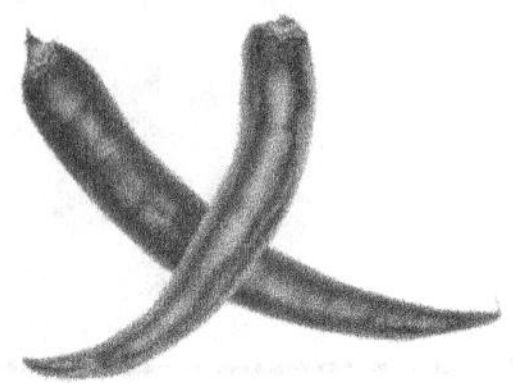

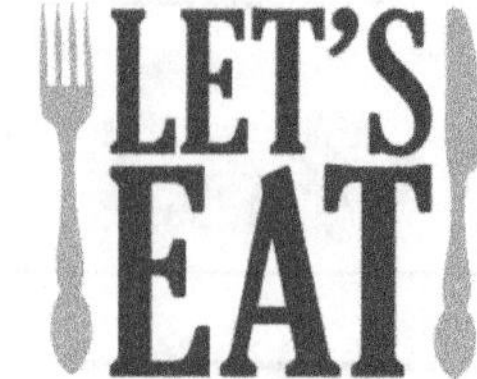

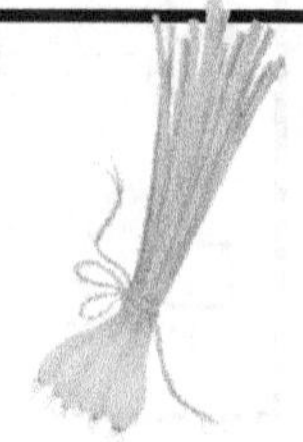

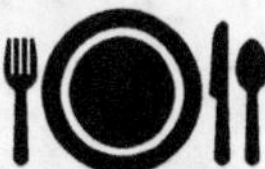 # Daily Healthy Eating Habits 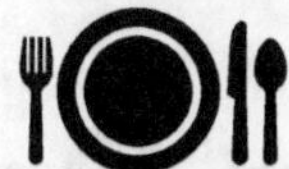

	Morning or Breakfast	Mid Day Or Lunch	Late Afternoon or Dinner	Evening Or Snacks
WATER- Drink 8-10 glasses or 3 L through out the day				
Veggies & Fruits- try to eat 5 servings each day				
Protein- Eat a palm size at each meal				
Healthy Fats- Eat fingertip - thumb size at each meal				
Follow Hand Portion Sizes at each meal				
Listen to Hunger & Fullness Cues				
Eat Mindfully & Slowly- Follow the 20 min meal				
Stop eating starchy carbs at 7pm				
Followed the 80/20 or 90/10 rule				
Any skipped meals				

Daily Exercise Plan

Activity	Length of W/O	Weight	Reps	Sets	Speed	Distance	Calories Burned

My Daily Reflections

Date:

⭐ Top 3 Daily Goals ⭐

- ☐ _______________________________
- ☐ _______________________________
- ☐ _______________________________

My Action Steps To Help Me Reach My Daily Goals Are:

♥ My Top 3 Strengths Are ♥

- ☐ _______________________________
- ☐ _______________________________
- ☐ _______________________________

Today I Found Happiness In

3 Things I Love About My Body

- ☐ _______________________________
- ☐ _______________________________
- ☐ _______________________________

I Am Grateful For

Daily Meal Planner

MEAL PLAN		Macros Counts
Breakfast		Calories______ Carbs:_______ Protein:______ Fats:________
Mid Morning		Calories______ Carbs:_______ Protein:______ Fats:________
Lunch		Calories______ Carbs:_______ Protein:______ Fats:________
Afternoon		Calories______ Carbs:_______ Protein:______ Fats:________
Dinner		Calories______ Carbs:_______ Protein:______ Fats:________

	Calories	Carbs	Protein	Fats
Calculated Macros				
Daily Totals				

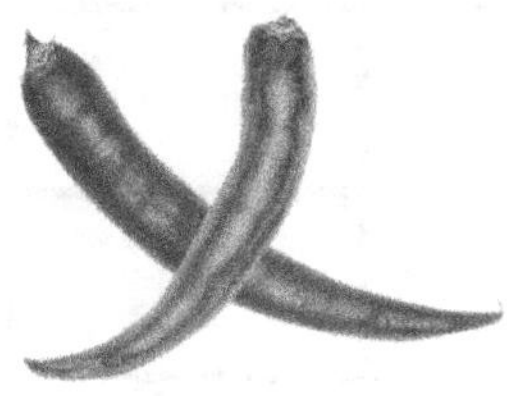

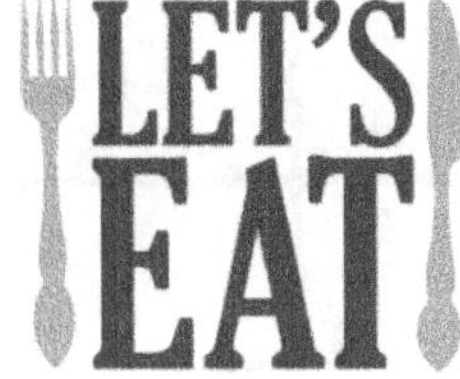

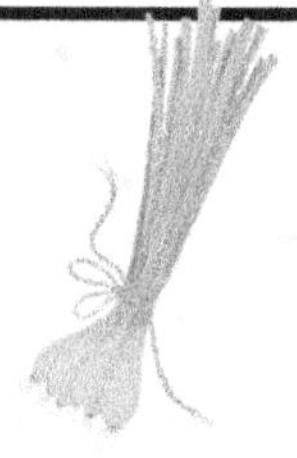

Daily Healthy Eating Habits

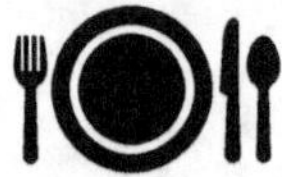 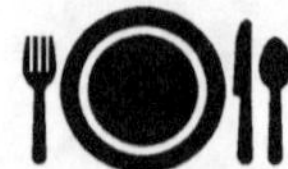

	Morning or Breakfast	Mid Day Or Lunch	Late Afternoon or Dinner	Evening Or Snacks
WATER- Drink 8-10 glasses or 3 L through out the day				
Veggies & Fruits- try to eat 5 servings each day				
Protein- Eat a palm size at each meal				
Healthy Fats- Eat fingertip - thumb size at each meal				
Follow Hand Portion Sizes at each meal				
Listen to Hunger & Fullness Cues				
Eat Mindfully & Slowly- Follow the 20 min meal				
Stop eating starchy carbs at 7pm				
Followed the 80/20 or 90/10 rule				
Any skipped meals				

Daily Exercise Plan

Activity	Length of W/O	Weight	Reps	Sets	Speed	Distance	Calories Burned

My Daily Reflections

Date:

Top 3 Daily Goals

- [ ] __________________________________
- [ ] __________________________________
- [ ] __________________________________

My Action Steps To Help Me Reach My Daily Goals Are:

My Top 3 Strengths Are

- [ ] __________________________________
- [ ] __________________________________
- [ ] __________________________________

Today I Found Happiness In

3 Things I Love About My Body

- [ ] __________________________________
- [ ] __________________________________
- [ ] __________________________________

I Am Grateful For

Daily Meal Planner

MEAL PLAN		Macros Counts
Breakfast		Calories_______ Carbs:_______ Protein:_______ Fats:_________
Mid Morning		Calories_______ Carbs:_______ Protein:_______ Fats:_________
Lunch		Calories_______ Carbs:_______ Protein:_______ Fats:_________
Afternoon		Calories_______ Carbs:_______ Protein:_______ Fats:_________
Dinner		Calories_______ Carbs:_______ Protein:_______ Fats:_________

	Calories	Carbs	Protein	Fats
Calculated Macros				
Daily Totals				

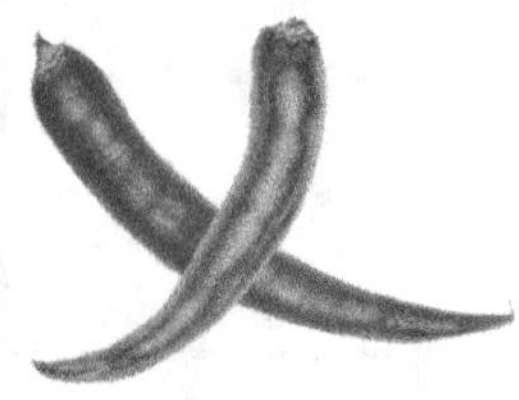
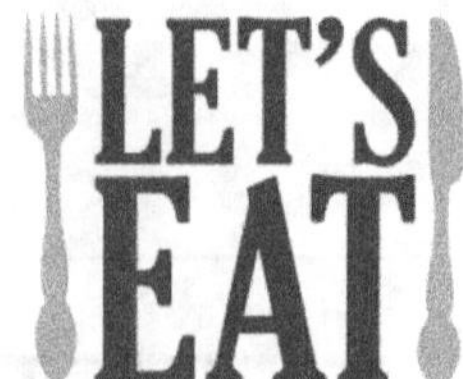

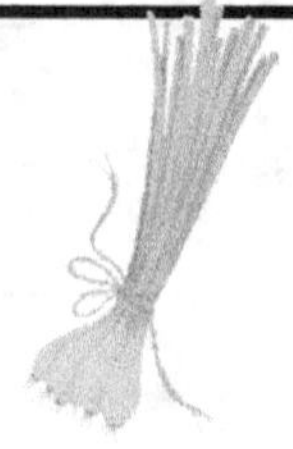

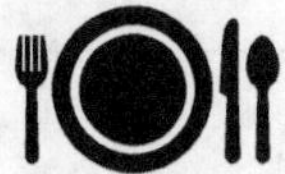 # Daily Healthy Eating Habits 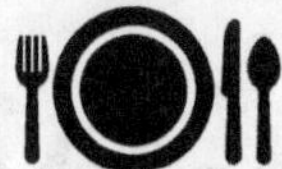

	Morning or Breakfast	Mid Day Or Lunch	Late Afternoon or Dinner	Evening Or Snacks
WATER- Drink 8-10 glasses or 3 L through out the day				
Veggies & Fruits- try to eat 5 servings each day				
Protein- Eat a palm size at each meal				
Healthy Fats- Eat fingertip - thumb size at each meal				
Follow Hand Portion Sizes at each meal				
Listen to Hunger & Fullness Cues				
Eat Mindfully & Slowly- Follow the 20 min meal				
Stop eating starchy carbs at 7pm				
Followed the 80/20 or 90/10 rule				
Any skipped meals				

Daily Exercise Plan

Activity	Length of W/O	Weight	Reps	Sets	Speed	Distance	Calories Burned

My Daily Reflections

Date:

⭐ Top 3 Daily Goals ⭐

☐ ______________________________

☐ ______________________________

☐ ______________________________

My Action Steps To Help Me Reach My Daily Goals Are:

♥ My Top 3 Strengths Are ♥

☐ ______________________________

☐ ______________________________

☐ ______________________________

Today I Found Happiness In

3 Things I Love About My Body

☐ ______________________________

☐ ______________________________

☐ ______________________________

I Am Grateful For

Daily Meal Planner

MEAL PLAN		Macros Counts
Breakfast		Calories______ Carbs:______ Protein:______ Fats:________
Mid Morning		Calories______ Carbs:______ Protein:______ Fats:________
Lunch		Calories______ Carbs:______ Protein:______ Fats:________
Afternoon		Calories______ Carbs:______ Protein:______ Fats:________
Dinner		Calories______ Carbs:______ Protein:______ Fats:________

	Calories	Carbs	Protein	Fats
Calculated Macros				
Daily Totals				

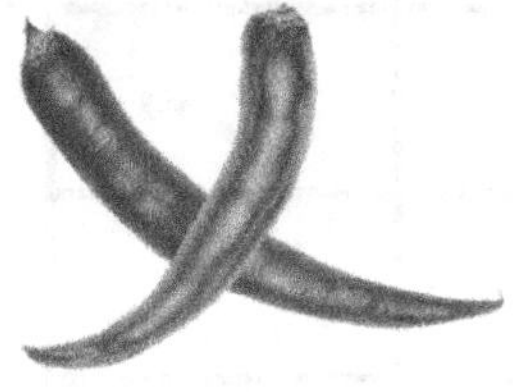

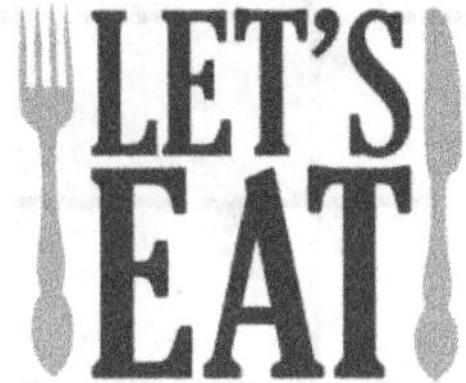

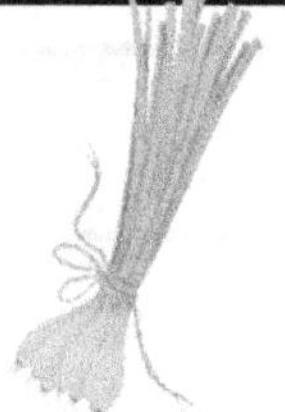

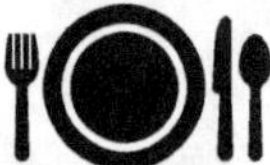 # Daily Healthy Eating Habits 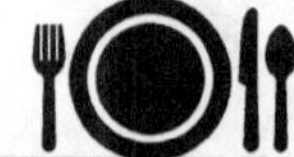

	Morning or Breakfast	Mid Day Or Lunch	Late Afternoon or Dinner	Evening Or Snacks
WATER- Drink 8-10 glasses or 3 L through out the day				
Veggies & Fruits- try to eat 5 servings each day				
Protein- Eat a palm size at each meal				
Healthy Fats- Eat fingertip - thumb size at each meal				
Follow Hand Portion Sizes at each meal				
Listen to Hunger & Fullness Cues				
Eat Mindfully & Slowly- Follow the 20 min meal				
Stop eating starchy carbs at 7pm				
Followed the 80/20 or 90/10 rule				
Any skipped meals				

Daily Exercise Plan

Activity	Length of W/O	Weight	Reps	Sets	Speed	Distance	Calories Burned

My Daily Reflections

Date:

⭐ Top 3 Daily Goals ⭐

My Action Steps To Help Me
Reach My Daily Goals Are:

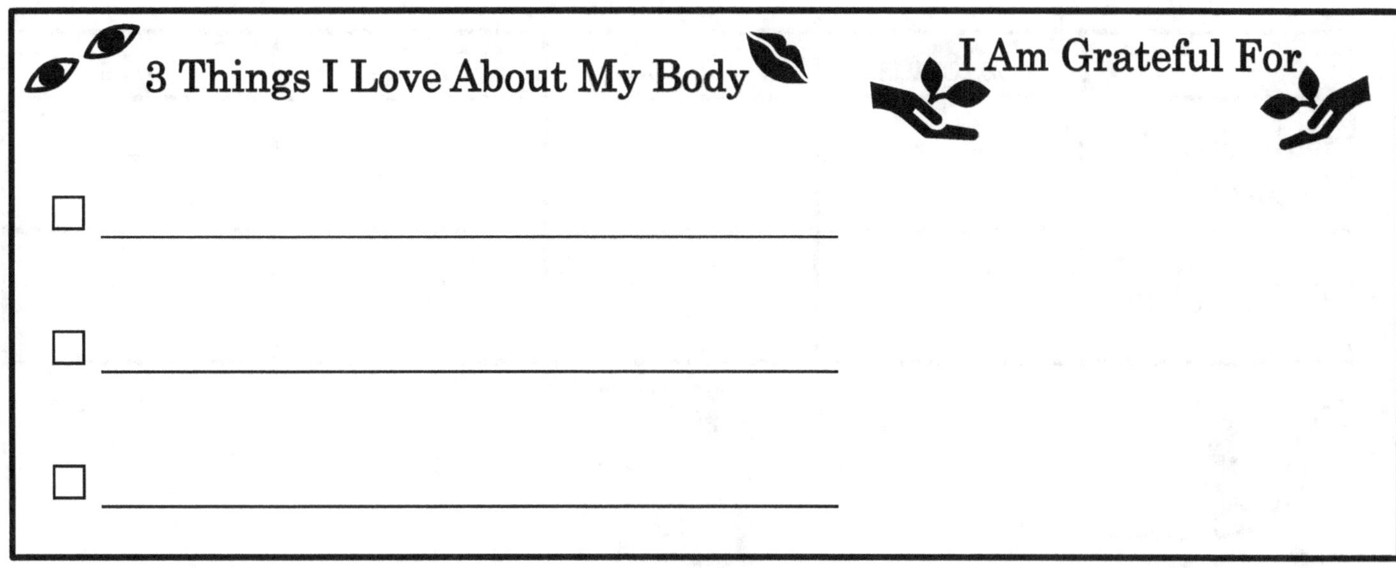

- ☐ _______________________
- ☐ _______________________
- ☐ _______________________

♥ My Top 3 Strengths Are ♥

Today I Found Happiness In

- ☐ _______________________
- ☐ _______________________
- ☐ _______________________

👀 3 Things I Love About My Body 💋

I Am Grateful For

- ☐ _______________________
- ☐ _______________________
- ☐ _______________________

Daily Meal Planner

MEAL PLAN		Macros Counts
Breakfast		Calories________ Carbs:________ Protein:______ Fats:__________
Mid Morning		Calories________ Carbs:________ Protein:______ Fats:__________
Lunch		Calories________ Carbs:________ Protein:______ Fats:__________
Afternoon		Calories________ Carbs:________ Protein:______ Fats:__________
Dinner		Calories________ Carbs:________ Protein:______ Fats:__________

	Calories	Carbs	Protein	Fats
Calculated Macros				
Daily Totals				

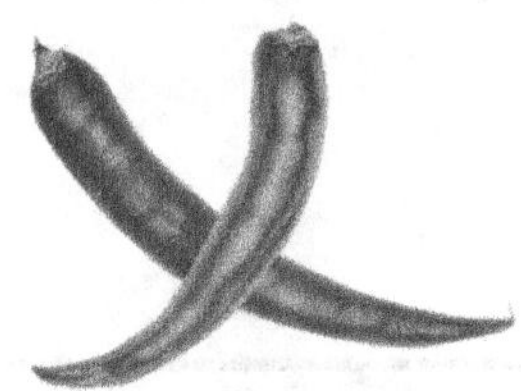
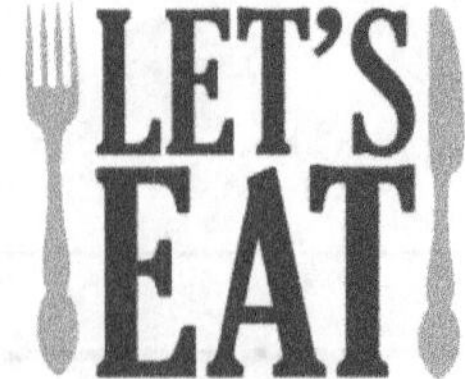

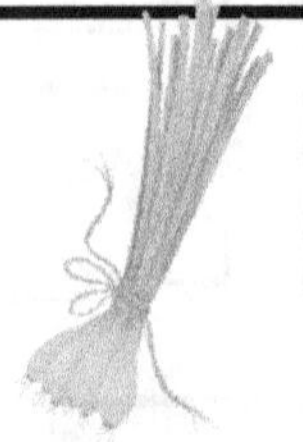

Daily Healthy Eating Habits

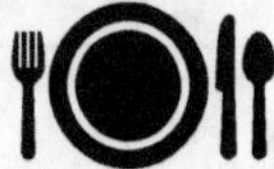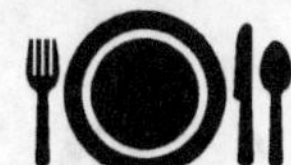

	Morning or Breakfast	Mid Day Or Lunch	Late Afternoon or Dinner	Evening Or Snacks
WATER- Drink 8-10 glasses or 3 L through out the day				
Veggies & Fruits- try to eat 5 servings each day				
Protein- Eat a palm size at each meal				
Healthy Fats- Eat fingertip - thumb size at each meal				
Follow Hand Portion Sizes at each meal				
Listen to Hunger & Fullness Cues				
Eat Mindfully & Slowly- Follow the 20 min meal				
Stop eating starchy carbs at 7pm				
Followed the 80/20 or 90/10 rule				
Any skipped meals				

Daily Exercise Plan

Activity	Length of W/O	Weight	Reps	Sets	Speed	Distance	Calories Burned

My Daily Reflections

Date:

Top 3 Daily Goals

☐ _______________________________

☐ _______________________________

☐ _______________________________

My Action Steps To Help Me Reach My Daily Goals Are:

My Top 3 Strengths Are

☐ _______________________________

☐ _______________________________

☐ _______________________________

Today I Found Happiness In

3 Things I Love About My Body

☐ _______________________________

☐ _______________________________

☐ _______________________________

I Am Grateful For

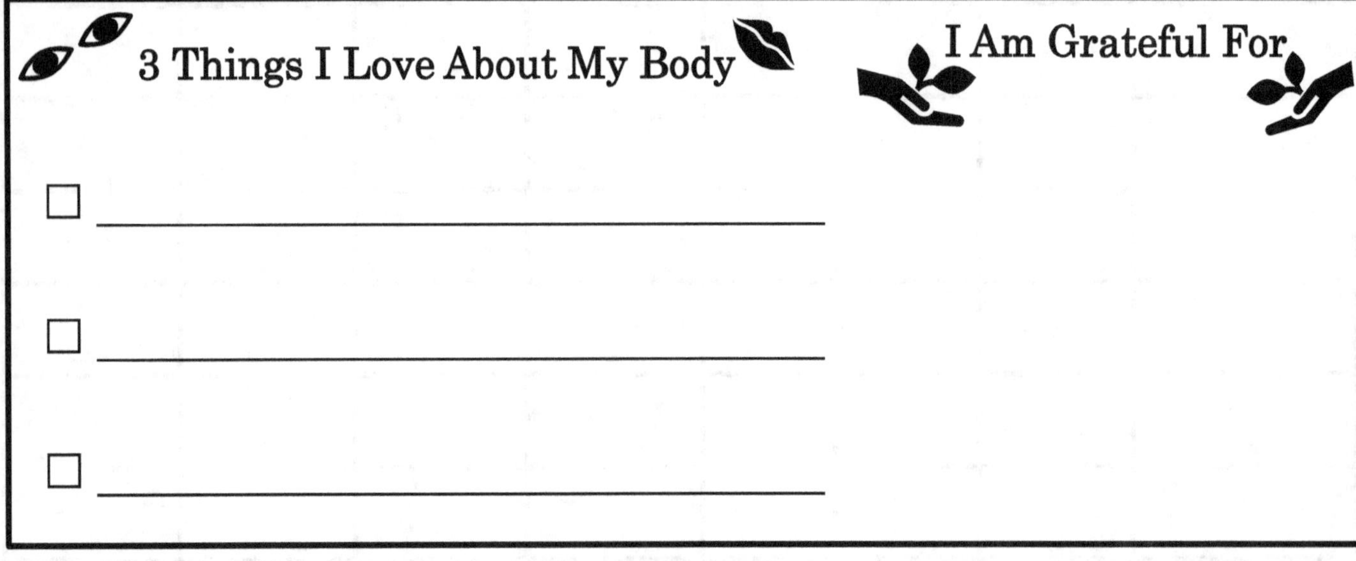

Daily Meal Planner

MEAL PLAN		Macros Counts
Breakfast		Calories________ Carbs:________ Protein:________ Fats:________
Mid Morning		Calories________ Carbs:________ Protein:________ Fats:________
Lunch		Calories________ Carbs:________ Protein:________ Fats:________
Afternoon		Calories________ Carbs:________ Protein:________ Fats:________
Dinner		Calories________ Carbs:________ Protein:________ Fats:________

	Calories	Carbs	Protein	Fats
Calculated Macros				
Daily Totals				

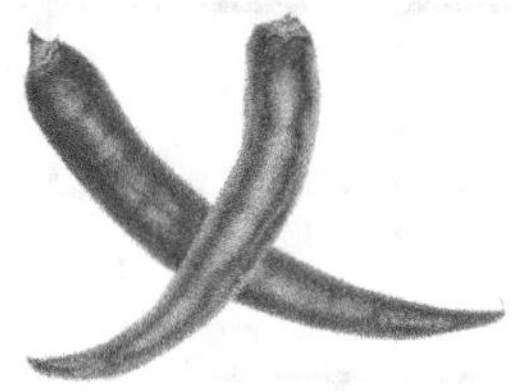

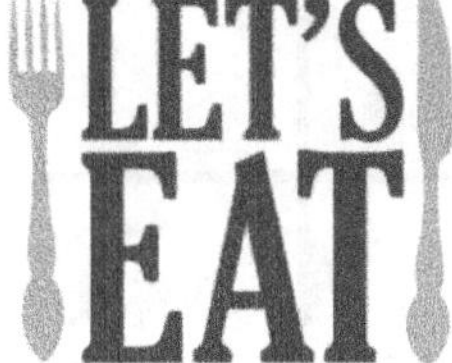

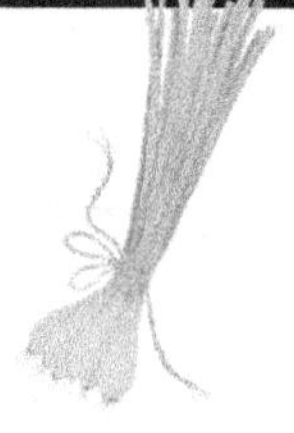

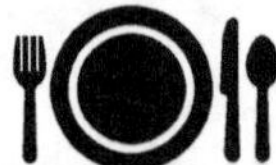 # Daily Healthy Eating Habits 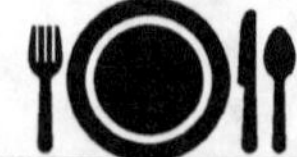

	Morning or Breakfast	Mid Day Or Lunch	Late Afternoon or Dinner	Evening Or Snacks
WATER- Drink 8-10 glasses or 3 L through out the day				
Veggies & Fruits- try to eat 5 servings each day				
Protein- Eat a palm size at each meal				
Healthy Fats- Eat fingertip - thumb size at each meal				
Follow Hand Portion Sizes at each meal				
Listen to Hunger & Fullness Cues				
Eat Mindfully & Slowly- Follow the 20 min meal				
Stop eating starchy carbs at 7pm				
Followed the 80/20 or 90/10 rule				
Any skipped meals				

Daily Exercise Plan

Activity	Length of W/O	Weight	Reps	Sets	Speed	Distance	Calories Burned

| Week Of: | 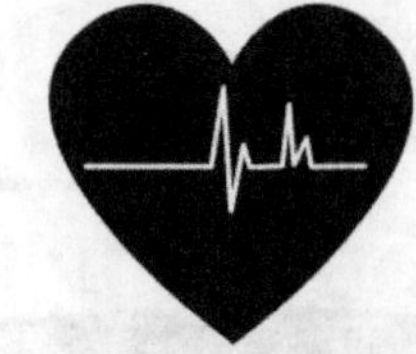 | | Track Your Blood Sugar | | |

Date	Wake Up	Pre-Lunch	Afternoon	Pre-Dinner	Bedtime

Results				
High				
Good				
Low				

Note Any Changes

WEEK 6 FROM: _______________

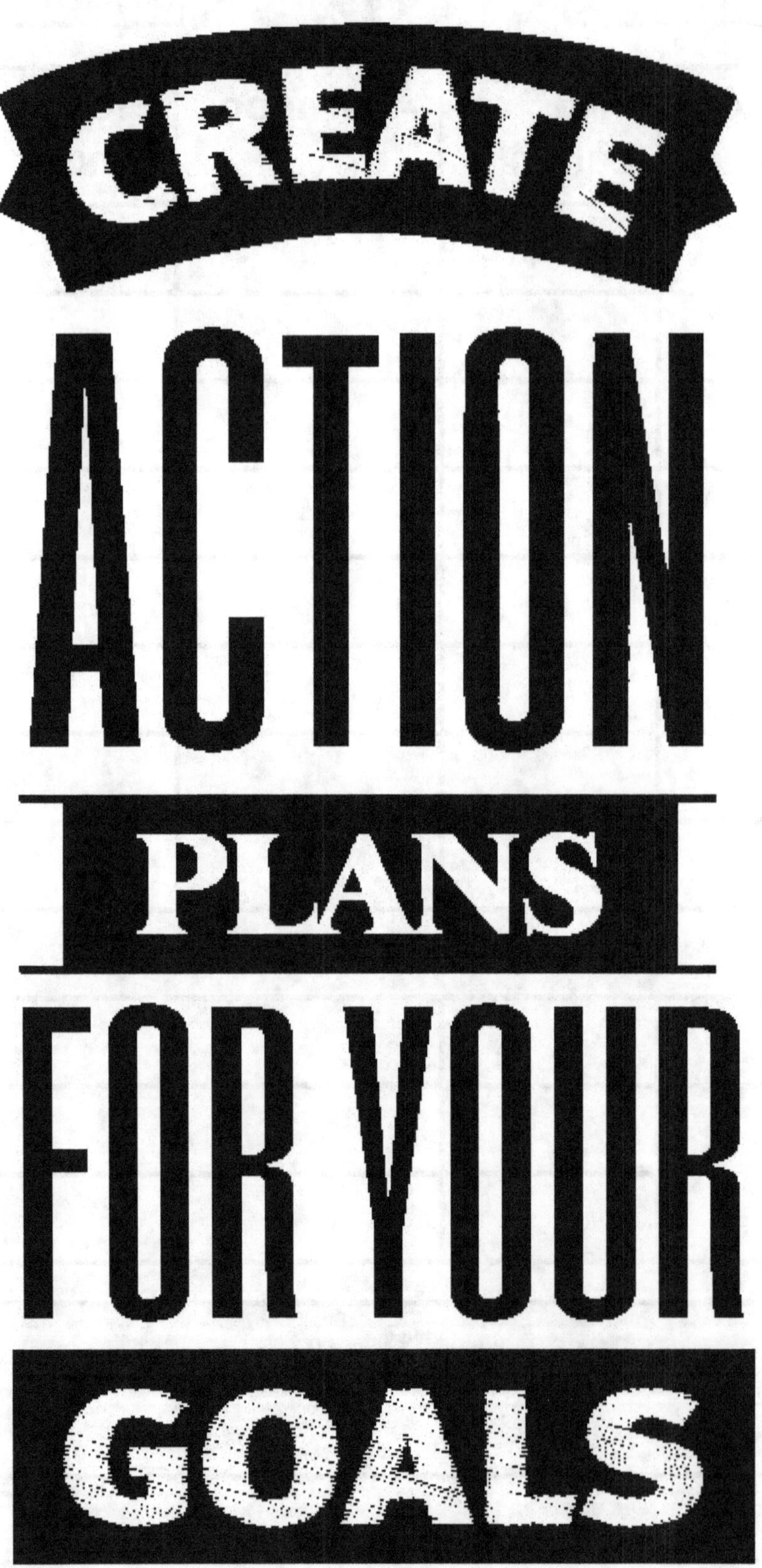

The Freedom of Self-Discipline

My Daily Reflections

Date:

⭐ Top 3 Daily Goals ⭐

- [ ] ______________________________
- [ ] ______________________________
- [ ] ______________________________

My Action Steps To Help Me Reach My Daily Goals Are:

❤ My Top 3 Strengths Are ❤

- [ ] ______________________________
- [ ] ______________________________
- [ ] ______________________________

Today I Found Happiness In

3 Things I Love About My Body

- [ ] ______________________________
- [ ] ______________________________
- [ ] ______________________________

I Am Grateful For

Daily Meal Planner

MEAL PLAN		Macros Counts
Breakfast		Calories________ Carbs:________ Protein:______ Fats:__________
Mid Morning		Calories________ Carbs:________ Protein:______ Fats:__________
Lunch		Calories________ Carbs:________ Protein:______ Fats:__________
Afternoon		Calories________ Carbs:________ Protein:______ Fats:__________
Dinner		Calories________ Carbs:________ Protein:______ Fats:__________

	Calories	Carbs	Protein	Fats
Calculated Macros				
Daily Totals				

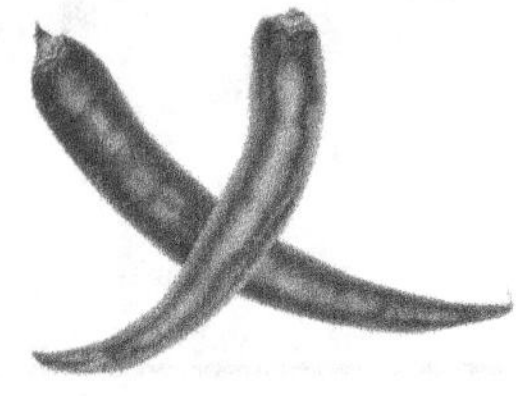

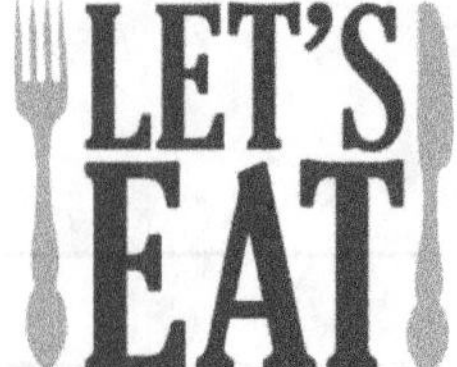

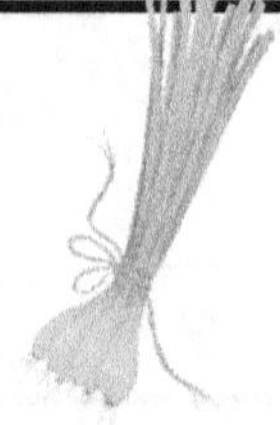

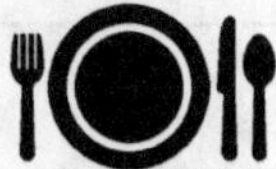 # Daily Healthy Eating Habits 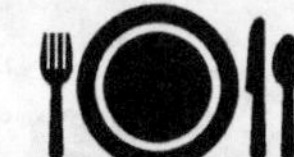

	Morning or Breakfast	Mid Day Or Lunch	Late Afternoon or Dinner	Evening Or Snacks
WATER- Drink 8-10 glasses or 3 L through out the day				
Veggies & Fruits- try to eat 5 servings each day				
Protein- Eat a palm size at each meal				
Healthy Fats- Eat fingertip - thumb size at each meal				
Follow Hand Portion Sizes at each meal				
Listen to Hunger & Fullness Cues				
Eat Mindfully & Slowly- Follow the 20 min meal				
Stop eating starchy carbs at 7pm				
Followed the 80/20 or 90/10 rule				
Any skipped meals				

Daily Exercise Plan

Activity	Length of W/O	Weight	Reps	Sets	Speed	Distance	Calories Burned

My Daily Reflections

Date:

Top 3 Daily Goals

- ☐ _______________________
- ☐ _______________________
- ☐ _______________________

My Action Steps To Help Me Reach My Daily Goals Are:

My Top 3 Strengths Are

- ☐ _______________________
- ☐ _______________________
- ☐ _______________________

Today I Found Happiness In

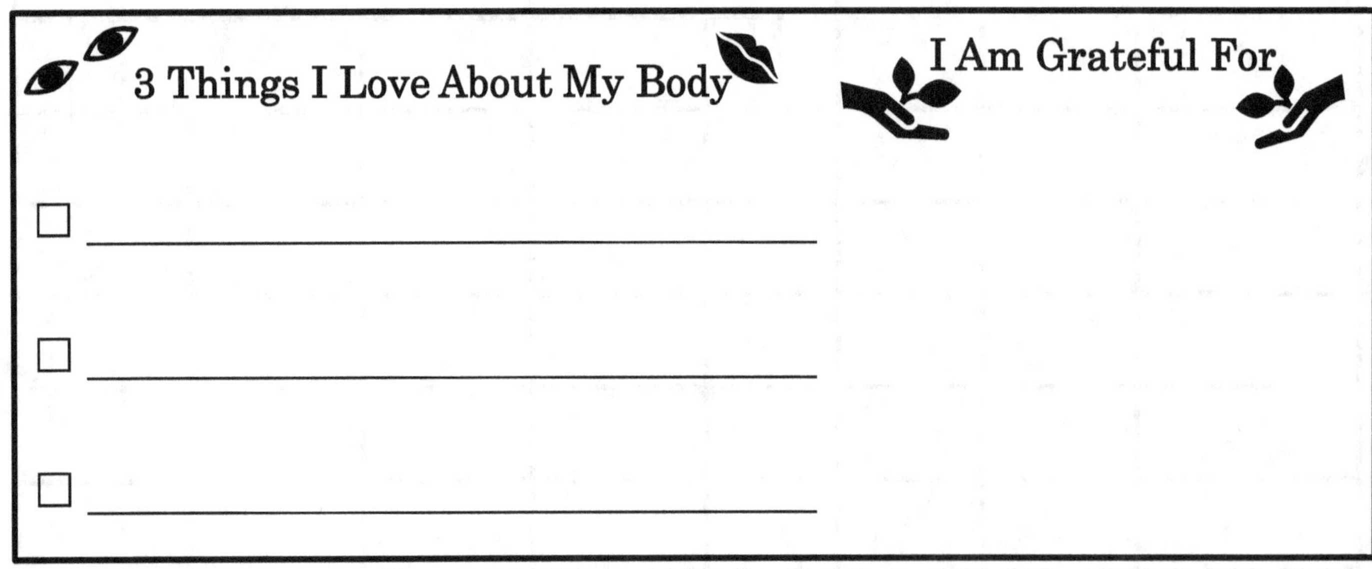

3 Things I Love About My Body

- ☐ _______________________
- ☐ _______________________
- ☐ _______________________

I Am Grateful For

Daily Meal Planner

MEAL PLAN		Macros Counts
Breakfast		Calories_______ Carbs:_______ Protein:______ Fats:_________
Mid Morning		Calories_______ Carbs:_______ Protein:______ Fats:_________
Lunch		Calories_______ Carbs:_______ Protein:______ Fats:_________
Afternoon		Calories_______ Carbs:_______ Protein:______ Fats:_________
Dinner		Calories_______ Carbs:_______ Protein:______ Fats:_________

	Calories	Carbs	Protein	Fats
Calculated Macros				
Daily Totals				

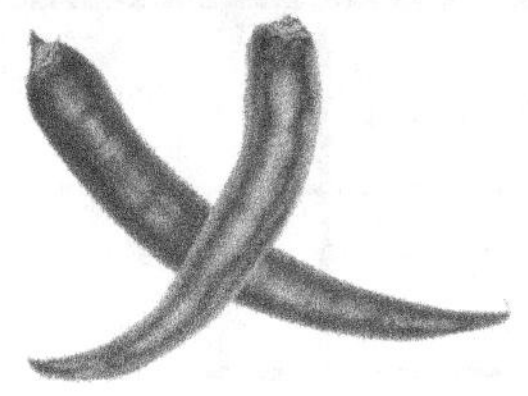

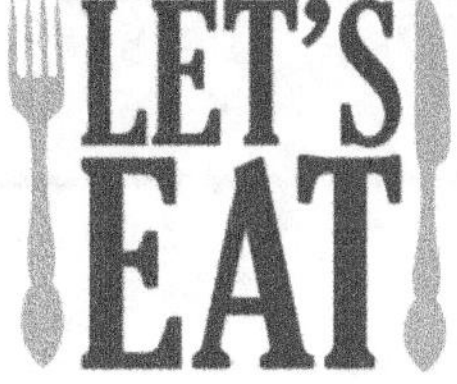

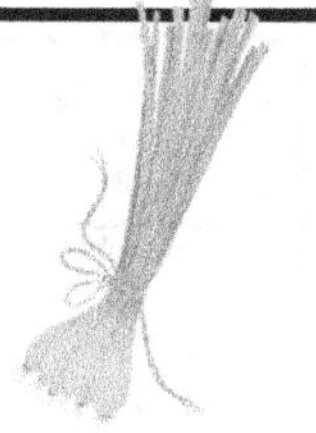

Daily Healthy Eating Habits

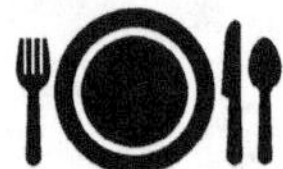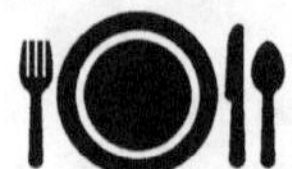

	Morning or Breakfast	Mid Day Or Lunch	Late Afternoon or Dinner	Evening Or Snacks
WATER- Drink 8-10 glasses or 3 L through out the day				
Veggies & Fruits- try to eat 5 servings each day				
Protein- Eat a palm size at each meal				
Healthy Fats- Eat fingertip - thumb size at each meal				
Follow Hand Portion Sizes at each meal				
Listen to Hunger & Fullness Cues				
Eat Mindfully & Slowly- Follow the 20 min meal				
Stop eating starchy carbs at 7pm				
Followed the 80/20 or 90/10 rule				
Any skipped meals				

Daily Exercise Plan

Activity	Length of W/O	Weight	Reps	Sets	Speed	Distance	Calories Burned

My Daily Reflections

Date:

★ Top 3 Daily Goals ★

☐ _______________

☐ _______________

☐ _______________

My Action Steps To Help Me Reach My Daily Goals Are:

♥ My Top 3 Strengths Are ♥

☐ _______________

☐ _______________

☐ _______________

Today I Found Happiness In

3 Things I Love About My Body

☐ _______________

☐ _______________

☐ _______________

I Am Grateful For

Daily Meal Planner

MEAL PLAN		Macros Counts
Breakfast		Calories________ Carbs:________ Protein:________ Fats:__________
Mid Morning		Calories________ Carbs:________ Protein:________ Fats:__________
Lunch		Calories________ Carbs:________ Protein:________ Fats:__________
Afternoon		Calories________ Carbs:________ Protein:________ Fats:__________
Dinner		Calories________ Carbs:________ Protein:________ Fats:__________

	Calories	Carbs	Protein	Fats
Calculated Macros				
Daily Totals				

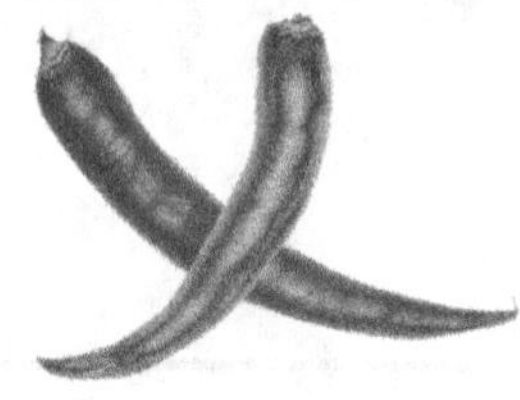

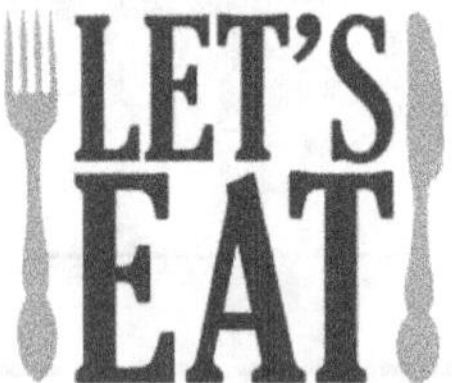

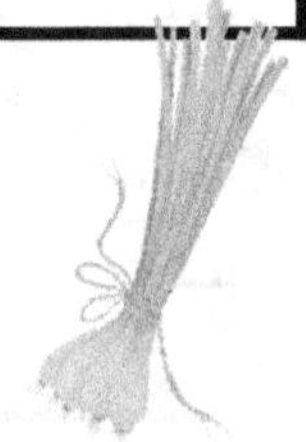

Daily Healthy Eating Habits

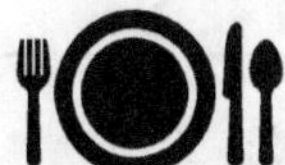
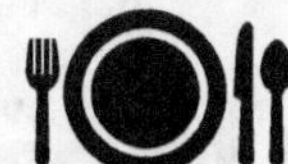

	Morning or Breakfast	Mid Day Or Lunch	Late Afternoon or Dinner	Evening Or Snacks
WATER- Drink 8-10 glasses or 3 L through out the day				
Veggies & Fruits- try to eat 5 servings each day				
Protein- Eat a palm size at each meal				
Healthy Fats- Eat fingertip - thumb size at each meal				
Follow Hand Portion Sizes at each meal				
Listen to Hunger & Fullness Cues				
Eat Mindfully & Slowly- Follow the 20 min meal				
Stop eating starchy carbs at 7pm				
Followed the 80/20 or 90/10 rule				
Any skipped meals				

Daily Exercise Plan

Activity	Length of W/O	Weight	Reps	Sets	Speed	Distance	Calories Burned

My Daily Reflections

Date:

★ Top 3 Daily Goals ★

☐ _______________________________

☐ _______________________________

☐ _______________________________

My Action Steps To Help Me Reach My Daily Goals Are:

♥ My Top 3 Strengths Are ♥

☐ _______________________________

☐ _______________________________

☐ _______________________________

Today I Found Happiness In

3 Things I Love About My Body

☐ _______________________________

☐ _______________________________

☐ _______________________________

I Am Grateful For

Daily Meal Planner

MEAL PLAN		Macros Counts
Breakfast		Calories______ Carbs:______ Protein:______ Fats:________
Mid Morning		Calories______ Carbs:______ Protein:______ Fats:________
Lunch		Calories______ Carbs:______ Protein:______ Fats:________
Afternoon		Calories______ Carbs:______ Protein:______ Fats:________
Dinner		Calories______ Carbs:______ Protein:______ Fats:________

	Calories	Carbs	Protein	Fats
Calculated Macros				
Daily Totals				

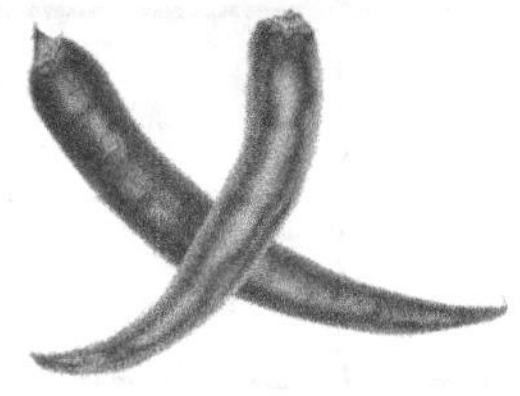
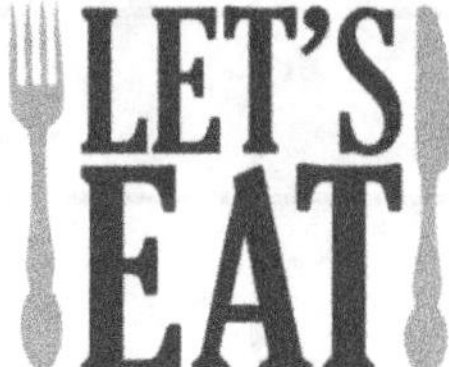

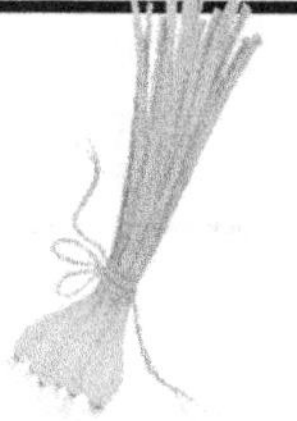

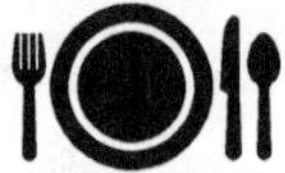 # Daily Healthy Eating Habits 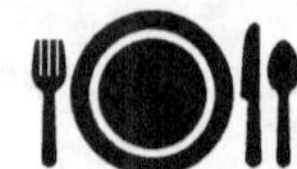

	Morning or Breakfast	Mid Day Or Lunch	Late Afternoon or Dinner	Evening Or Snacks
WATER- Drink 8-10 glasses or 3 L through out the day				
Veggies & Fruits- try to eat 5 servings each day				
Protein- Eat a palm size at each meal				
Healthy Fats- Eat fingertip - thumb size at each meal				
Follow Hand Portion Sizes at each meal				
Listen to Hunger & Fullness Cues				
Eat Mindfully & Slowly- Follow the 20 min meal				
Stop eating starchy carbs at 7pm				
Followed the 80/20 or 90/10 rule				
Any skipped meals				

Daily Exercise Plan

Activity	Length of W/O	Weight	Reps	Sets	Speed	Distance	Calories Burned

My Daily Reflections

Date:

Top 3 Daily Goals

My Action Steps To Help Me
Reach My Daily Goals Are:

My Top 3 Strengths Are

Today I Found Happiness In

3 Things I Love About My Body

I Am Grateful For

Daily Meal Planner

MEAL PLAN		Macros Counts
Breakfast		Calories______ Carbs:______ Protein:______ Fats:________
Mid Morning		Calories______ Carbs:______ Protein:______ Fats:________
Lunch		Calories______ Carbs:______ Protein:______ Fats:________
Afternoon		Calories______ Carbs:______ Protein:______ Fats:________
Dinner		Calories______ Carbs:______ Protein:______ Fats:________

	Calories	Carbs	Protein	Fats
Calculated Macros				
Daily Totals				

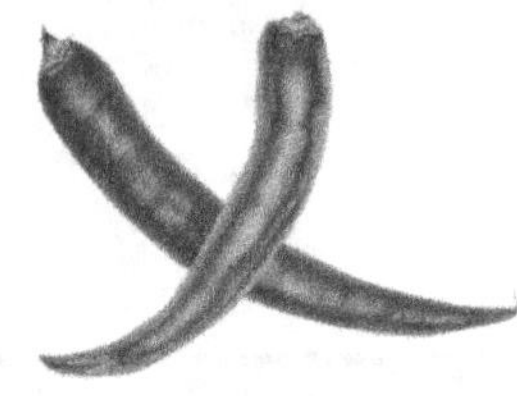

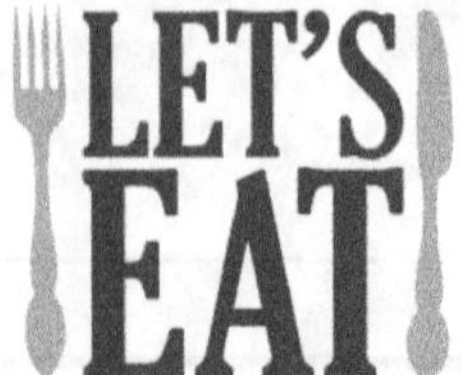

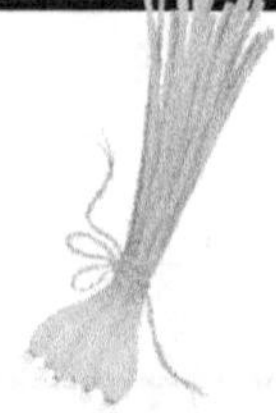

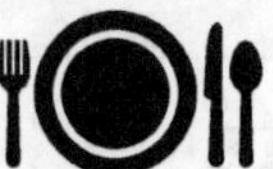 Daily Healthy Eating Habits 

	Morning or Breakfast	Mid Day Or Lunch	Late Afternoon or Dinner	Evening Or Snacks
WATER- Drink 8-10 glasses or 3 L through out the day				
Veggies & Fruits- try to eat 5 servings each day				
Protein- Eat a palm size at each meal				
Healthy Fats- Eat fingertip - thumb size at each meal				
Follow Hand Portion Sizes at each meal				
Listen to Hunger & Fullness Cues				
Eat Mindfully & Slowly- Follow the 20 min meal				
Stop eating starchy carbs at 7pm				
Followed the 80/20 or 90/10 rule				
Any skipped meals				

Daily Exercise Plan

Activity	Length of W/O	Weight	Reps	Sets	Speed	Distance	Calories Burned

My Daily Reflections

Date:

Top 3 Daily Goals

☐ __________________________

☐ __________________________

☐ __________________________

My Action Steps To Help Me Reach My Daily Goals Are:

My Top 3 Strengths Are

☐ __________________________

☐ __________________________

☐ __________________________

Today I Found Happiness In

3 Things I Love About My Body

☐ __________________________

☐ __________________________

☐ __________________________

I Am Grateful For

Daily Meal Planner

MEAL PLAN		Macros Counts
Breakfast		Calories________ Carbs:________ Protein:_______ Fats:__________
Mid Morning		Calories________ Carbs:________ Protein:_______ Fats:__________
Lunch		Calories________ Carbs:________ Protein:_______ Fats:__________
Afternoon		Calories________ Carbs:________ Protein:_______ Fats:__________
Dinner		Calories________ Carbs:________ Protein:_______ Fats:__________

	Calories	Carbs	Protein	Fats
Calculated Macros				
Daily Totals				

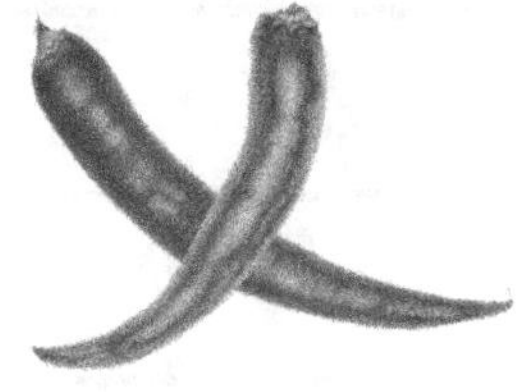

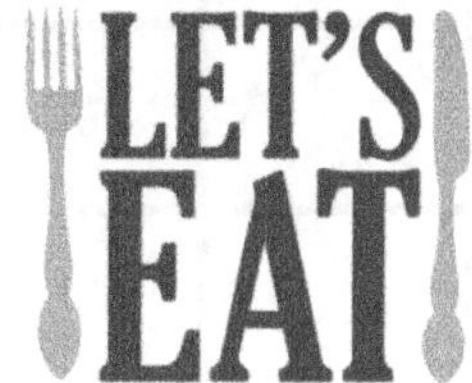

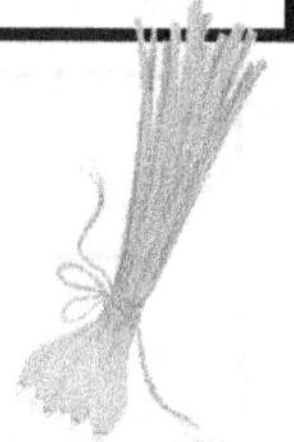

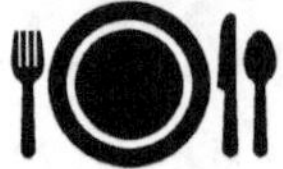 Daily Healthy Eating Habits 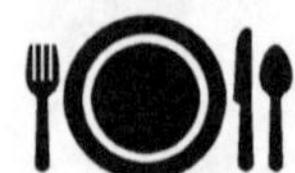

	Morning or Breakfast	Mid Day Or Lunch	Late Afternoon or Dinner	Evening Or Snacks
WATER- Drink 8-10 glasses or 3 L through out the day	○ ○ ○ ○ ○ ○ ○ ○			
Veggies & Fruits- try to eat 5 servings each day	🍎 🍎 🍎 🍎 🍎 🍎 🍎			
Protein- Eat a palm size at each meal				
Healthy Fats- Eat fingertip - thumb size at each meal				
Follow Hand Portion Sizes at each meal				
Listen to Hunger & Fullness Cues				
Eat Mindfully & Slowly- Follow the 20 min meal				
Stop eating starchy carbs at 7pm				
Followed the 80/20 or 90/10 rule				
Any skipped meals				

Daily Exercise Plan

Activity	Length of W/O	Weight	Reps	Sets	Speed	Distance	Calories Burned

My Daily Reflections

Date:

Top 3 Daily Goals

☐ ____

☐ ____

☐ ____

My Action Steps To Help Me Reach My Daily Goals Are:

My Top 3 Strengths Are

☐ ____

☐ ____

☐ ____

Today I Found Happiness In

3 Things I Love About My Body

☐ ____

☐ ____

☐ ____

I Am Grateful For

Daily Meal Planner

MEAL PLAN		Macros Counts
Breakfast		Calories______ Carbs:______ Protein:______ Fats:________
Mid Morning		Calories______ Carbs:______ Protein:______ Fats:________
Lunch		Calories______ Carbs:______ Protein:______ Fats:________
Afternoon		Calories______ Carbs:______ Protein:______ Fats:________
Dinner		Calories______ Carbs:______ Protein:______ Fats:________

	Calories	Carbs	Protein	Fats
Calculated Macros				
Daily Totals				

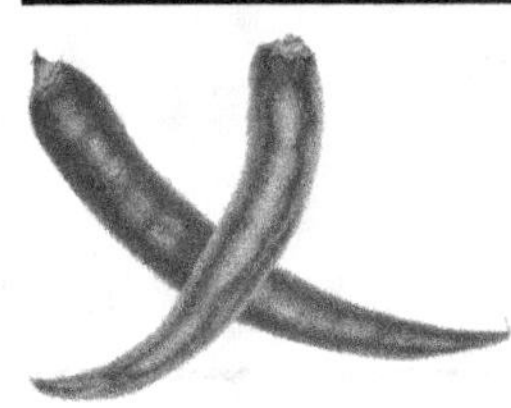

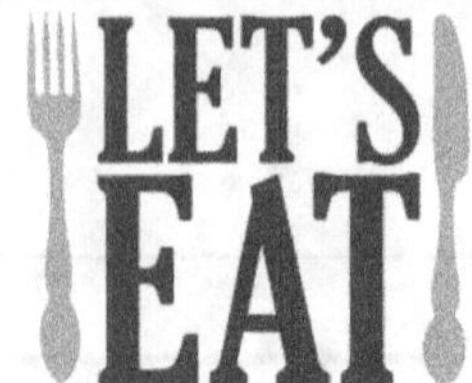

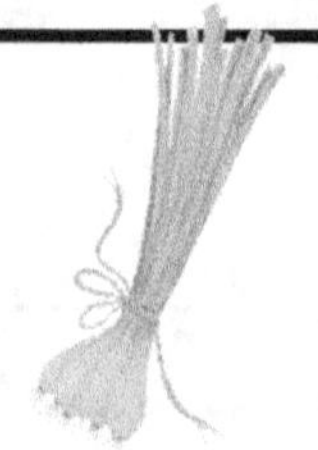

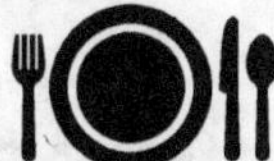 # Daily Healthy Eating Habits 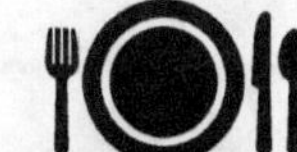

	Morning or Breakfast	Mid Day Or Lunch	Late Afternoon or Dinner	Evening Or Snacks
WATER- Drink 8-10 glasses or 3 L through out the day				
Veggies & Fruits- try to eat 5 servings each day				
Protein- Eat a palm size at each meal				
Healthy Fats- Eat fingertip - thumb size at each meal				
Follow Hand Portion Sizes at each meal				
Listen to Hunger & Fullness Cues				
Eat Mindfully & Slowly- Follow the 20 min meal				
Stop eating starchy carbs at 7pm				
Followed the 80/20 or 90/10 rule				
Any skipped meals				

Daily Exercise Plan

Activity	Length of W/O	Weight	Reps	Sets	Speed	Distance	Calories Burned

<table>
<tr><td>

Week Of:
</td><td>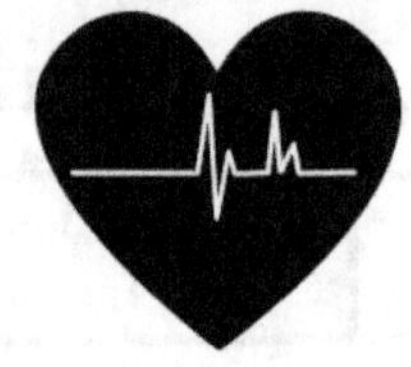</td><td>

Track Your Blood Sugar
</td></tr>
</table>

Date	Wake Up	Pre-Lunch	Afternoon	Pre-Dinner	Bedtime

Results

High					
Good					
Low					

Note Any Changes

WEEK 7 FROM:

STEP
OUTSIDE
YOUR COMFORT
ZONE

BEING MORE DARING

My Daily Reflections

Date:

Top 3 Daily Goals

☐ _______________________

☐ _______________________

☐ _______________________

My Action Steps To Help Me Reach My Daily Goals Are:

My Top 3 Strengths Are

☐ _______________________

☐ _______________________

☐ _______________________

Today I Found Happiness In

3 Things I Love About My Body

☐ _______________________

☐ _______________________

☐ _______________________

I Am Grateful For

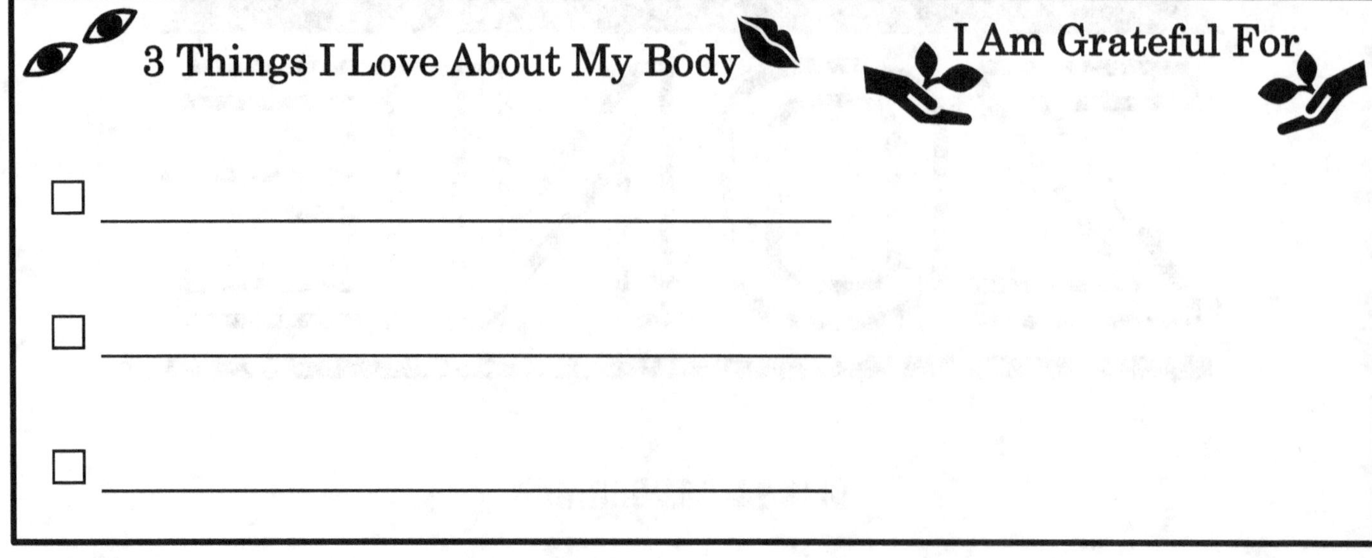

Daily Meal Planner

MEAL PLAN		Macros Counts
Breakfast		Calories______ Carbs:________ Protein:______ Fats:_________
Mid Morning		Calories______ Carbs:________ Protein:______ Fats:_________
Lunch		Calories______ Carbs:________ Protein:______ Fats:_________
Afternoon		Calories______ Carbs:________ Protein:______ Fats:_________
Dinner		Calories______ Carbs:________ Protein:______ Fats:_________

	Calories	Carbs	Protein	Fats
Calculated Macros				
Daily Totals				

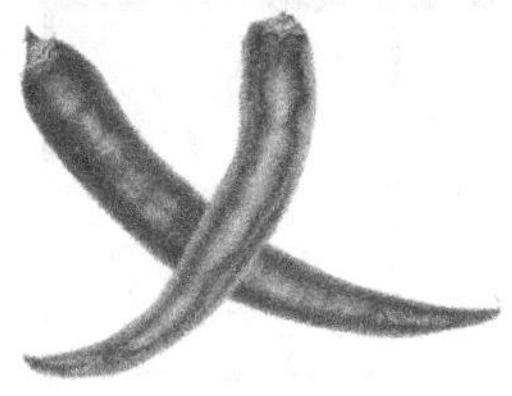

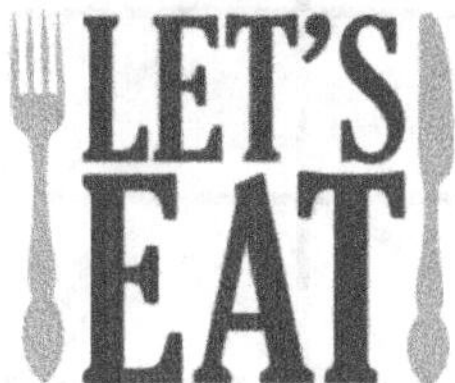

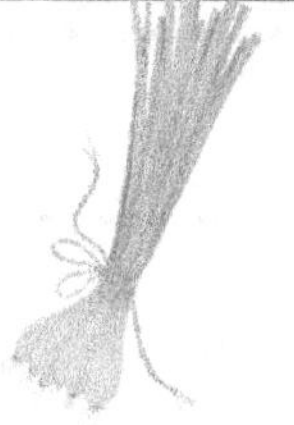

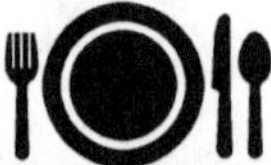# Daily Healthy Eating Habits 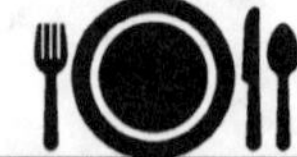

	Morning or Breakfast	Mid Day Or Lunch	Late Afternoon or Dinner	Evening Or Snacks
WATER- Drink 8-10 glasses or 3 L through out the day				
Veggies & Fruits- try to eat 5 servings each day				
Protein- Eat a palm size at each meal				
Healthy Fats- Eat fingertip - thumb size at each meal				
Follow Hand Portion Sizes at each meal				
Listen to Hunger & Fullness Cues				
Eat Mindfully & Slowly- Follow the 20 min meal				
Stop eating starchy carbs at 7pm				
Followed the 80/20 or 90/10 rule				
Any skipped meals				

Daily Exercise Plan

Activity	Length of W/O	Weight	Reps	Sets	Speed	Distance	Calories Burned

My Daily Reflections

Date:

Top 3 Daily Goals

My Action Steps To Help Me Reach My Daily Goals Are:

My Top 3 Strengths Are

Today I Found Happiness In

3 Things I Love About My Body

I Am Grateful For

Daily Meal Planner

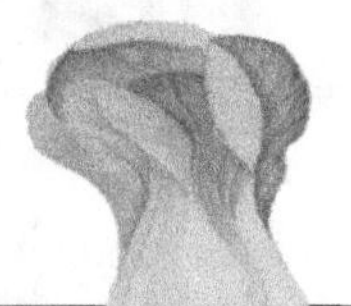

MEAL PLAN		Macros Counts
Breakfast		Calories________ Carbs:________ Protein:________ Fats:__________
Mid Morning		Calories________ Carbs:________ Protein:________ Fats:__________
Lunch		Calories________ Carbs:________ Protein:________ Fats:__________
Afternoon		Calories________ Carbs:________ Protein:________ Fats:__________
Dinner		Calories________ Carbs:________ Protein:________ Fats:__________

	Calories	Carbs	Protein	Fats
Calculated Macros				
Daily Totals				

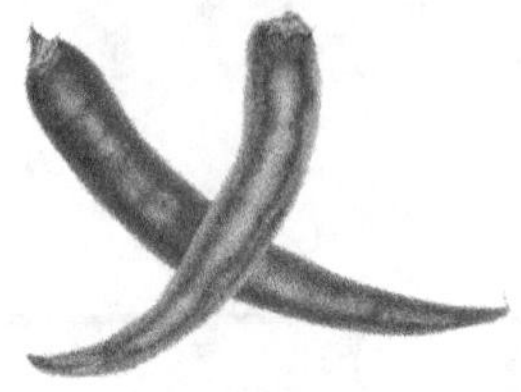

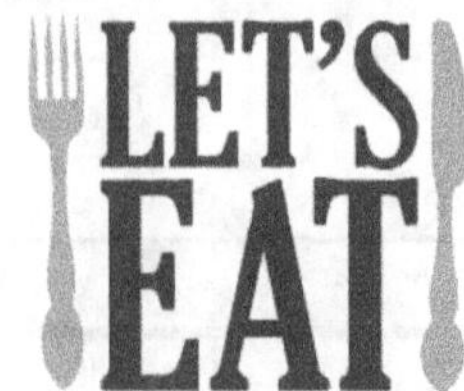

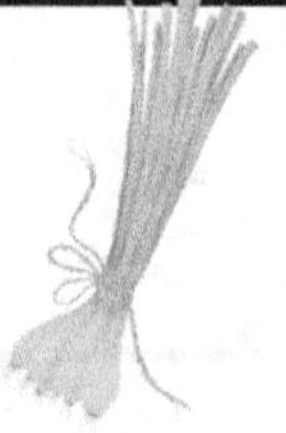

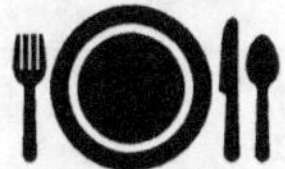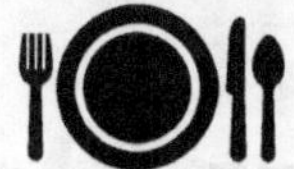

Daily Healthy Eating Habits

	Morning or Breakfast	Mid Day Or Lunch	Late Afternoon or Dinner	Evening Or Snacks
WATER- Drink 8-10 glasses or 3 L through out the day				
Veggies & Fruits- try to eat 5 servings each day				
Protein- Eat a palm size at each meal				
Healthy Fats- Eat fingertip - thumb size at each meal				
Follow Hand Portion Sizes at each meal				
Listen to Hunger & Fullness Cues				
Eat Mindfully & Slowly- Follow the 20 min meal				
Stop eating starchy carbs at 7pm				
Followed the 80/20 or 90/10 rule				
Any skipped meals				

Daily Exercise Plan

Activity	Length of W/O	Weight	Reps	Sets	Speed	Distance	Calories Burned

My Daily Reflections

Date:

⭐ Top 3 Daily Goals ⭐

☐ _______________________

☐ _______________________

☐ _______________________

My Action Steps To Help Me Reach My Daily Goals Are:

♥ My Top 3 Strengths Are ♥

☐ _______________________

☐ _______________________

☐ _______________________

Today I Found Happiness In

3 Things I Love About My Body

☐ _______________________

☐ _______________________

☐ _______________________

I Am Grateful For

Daily Meal Planner

MEAL PLAN		Macros Counts
Breakfast		Calories________ Carbs:________ Protein:______ Fats:________
Mid Morning		Calories________ Carbs:________ Protein:______ Fats:________
Lunch		Calories________ Carbs:________ Protein:______ Fats:________
Afternoon		Calories________ Carbs:________ Protein:______ Fats:________
Dinner		Calories________ Carbs:________ Protein:______ Fats:________

	Calories	Carbs	Protein	Fats
Calculated Macros				
Daily Totals				

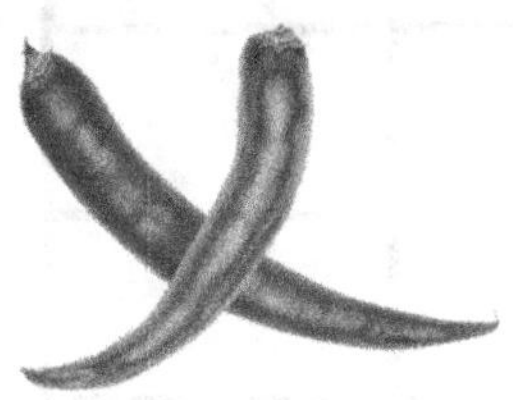

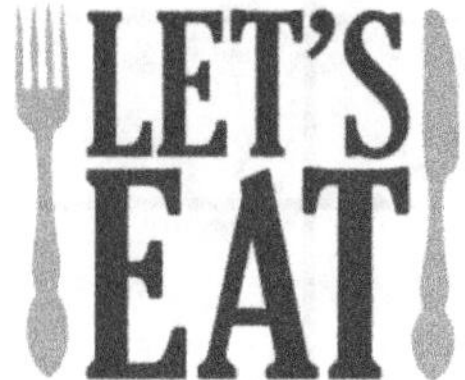

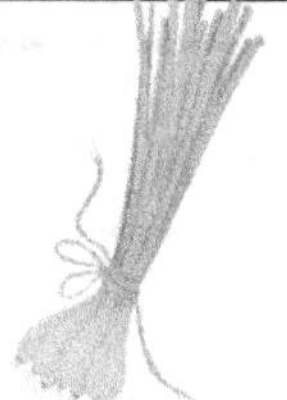

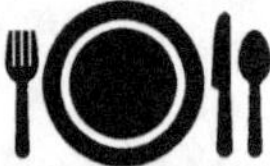 # Daily Healthy Eating Habits 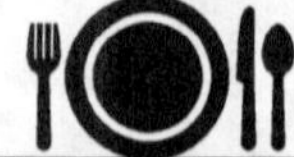

	Morning or Breakfast	Mid Day Or Lunch	Late Afternoon or Dinner	Evening Or Snacks
WATER- Drink 8-10 glasses or 3 L through out the day				
Veggies & Fruits- try to eat 5 servings each day				
Protein- Eat a palm size at each meal				
Healthy Fats- Eat fingertip - thumb size at each meal				
Follow Hand Portion Sizes at each meal				
Listen to Hunger & Fullness Cues				
Eat Mindfully & Slowly- Follow the 20 min meal				
Stop eating starchy carbs at 7pm				
Followed the 80/20 or 90/10 rule				
Any skipped meals				

Daily Exercise Plan

Activity	Length of W/O	Weight	Reps	Sets	Speed	Distance	Calories Burned

My Daily Reflections

Date:

Top 3 Daily Goals

My Action Steps To Help Me Reach My Daily Goals Are:

- ☐ ________________________
- ☐ ________________________
- ☐ ________________________

My Top 3 Strengths Are

Today I Found Happiness In

- ☐ ________________________
- ☐ ________________________
- ☐ ________________________

3 Things I Love About My Body

I Am Grateful For

- ☐ ________________________
- ☐ ________________________
- ☐ ________________________

Daily Meal Planner

MEAL PLAN	Macros Counts
Breakfast	Calories________ Carbs:________ Protein:________ Fats:__________
Mid Morning	Calories________ Carbs:________ Protein:________ Fats:__________
Lunch	Calories________ Carbs:________ Protein:________ Fats:__________
Afternoon	Calories________ Carbs:________ Protein:________ Fats:__________
Dinner	Calories________ Carbs:________ Protein:________ Fats:__________

	Calories	Carbs	Protein	Fats
Calculated Macros				
Daily Totals				

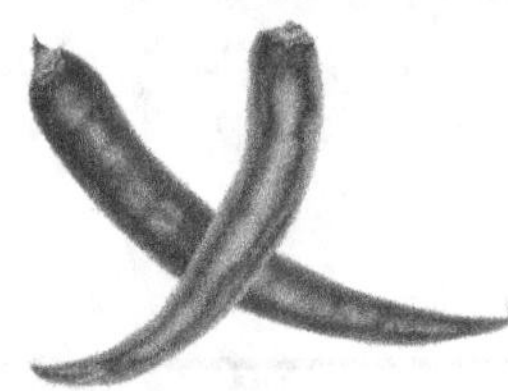

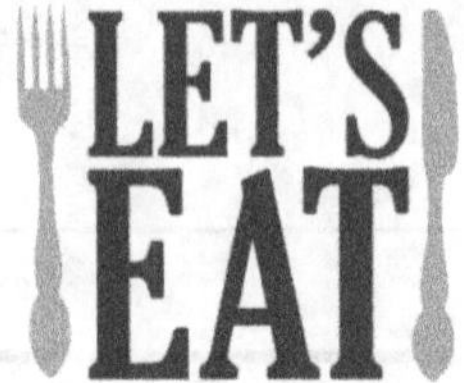

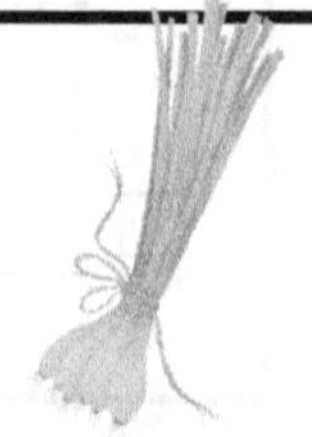

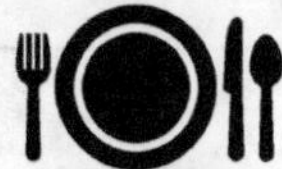 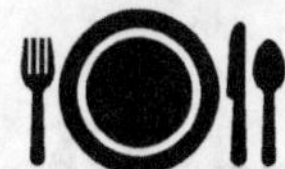

Daily Healthy Eating Habits

	Morning or Breakfast	Mid Day Or Lunch	Late Afternoon or Dinner	Evening Or Snacks
WATER- Drink 8-10 glasses or 3 L through out the day				
Veggies & Fruits- try to eat 5 servings each day				
Protein- Eat a palm size at each meal				
Healthy Fats- Eat fingertip - thumb size at each meal				
Follow Hand Portion Sizes at each meal				
Listen to Hunger & Fullness Cues				
Eat Mindfully & Slowly- Follow the 20 min meal				
Stop eating starchy carbs at 7pm				
Followed the 80/20 or 90/10 rule				
Any skipped meals				

Daily Exercise Plan

Activity	Length of W/O	Weight	Reps	Sets	Speed	Distance	Calories Burned

My Daily Reflections

Date:

Top 3 Daily Goals

☐ _______________________________

☐ _______________________________

☐ _______________________________

My Action Steps To Help Me Reach My Daily Goals Are:

My Top 3 Strengths Are

☐ _______________________________

☐ _______________________________

☐ _______________________________

Today I Found Happiness In

3 Things I Love About My Body

☐ _______________________________

☐ _______________________________

☐ _______________________________

I Am Grateful For

Daily Meal Planner

MEAL PLAN		Macros Counts
Breakfast		Calories________ Carbs:________ Protein:________ Fats:________
Mid Morning		Calories________ Carbs:________ Protein:________ Fats:________
Lunch		Calories________ Carbs:________ Protein:________ Fats:________
Afternoon		Calories________ Carbs:________ Protein:________ Fats:________
Dinner		Calories________ Carbs:________ Protein:________ Fats:________

	Calories	Carbs	Protein	Fats
Calculated Macros				
Daily Totals				

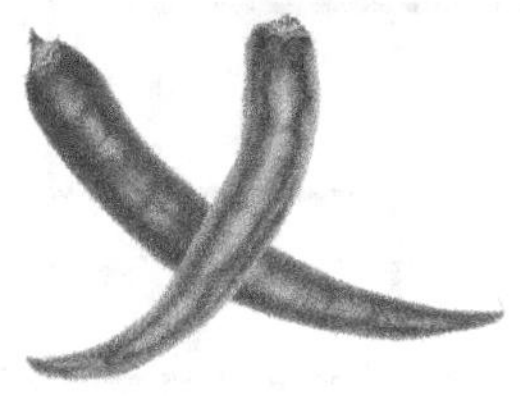

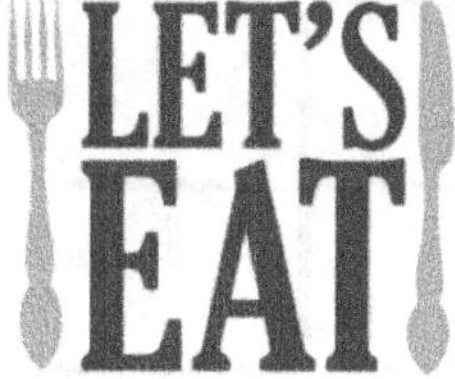

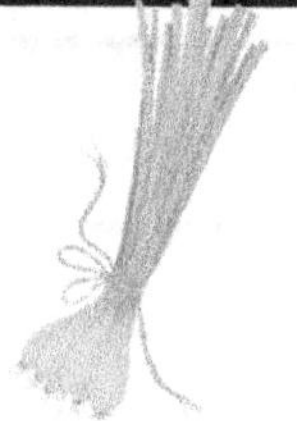

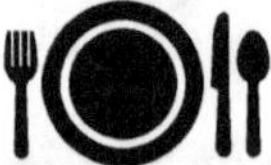 # Daily Healthy Eating Habits 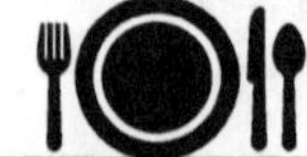

	Morning or Breakfast	Mid Day Or Lunch	Late Afternoon or Dinner	Evening Or Snacks
WATER- Drink 8-10 glasses or 3 L through out the day				
Veggies & Fruits- try to eat 5 servings each day				
Protein- Eat a palm size at each meal				
Healthy Fats- Eat fingertip - thumb size at each meal				
Follow Hand Portion Sizes at each meal				
Listen to Hunger & Fullness Cues				
Eat Mindfully & Slowly- Follow the 20 min meal				
Stop eating starchy carbs at 7pm				
Followed the 80/20 or 90/10 rule				
Any skipped meals				

Daily Exercise Plan

Activity	Length of W/O	Weight	Reps	Sets	Speed	Distance	Calories Burned

My Daily Reflections

Date:

Top 3 Daily Goals

My Action Steps To Help Me
Reach My Daily Goals Are:

My Top 3 Strengths Are

Today I Found Happiness In

3 Things I Love About My Body

I Am Grateful For

Daily Meal Planner

MEAL PLAN		Macros Counts
Breakfast		Calories______ Carbs:_______ Protein:______ Fats:________
Mid Morning		Calories______ Carbs:_______ Protein:______ Fats:________
Lunch		Calories______ Carbs:_______ Protein:______ Fats:________
Afternoon		Calories______ Carbs:_______ Protein:______ Fats:________
Dinner		Calories______ Carbs:_______ Protein:______ Fats:________

	Calories	Carbs	Protein	Fats
Calculated Macros				
Daily Totals				

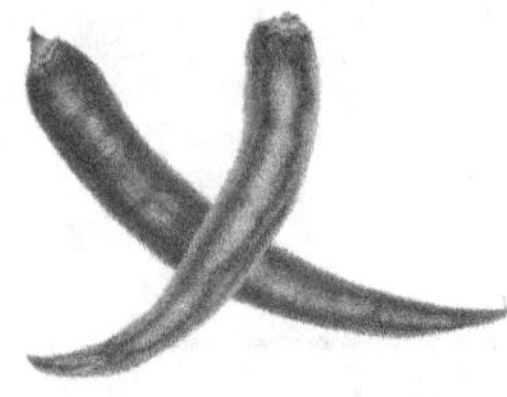
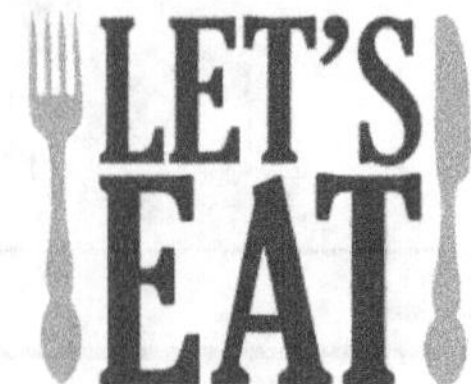

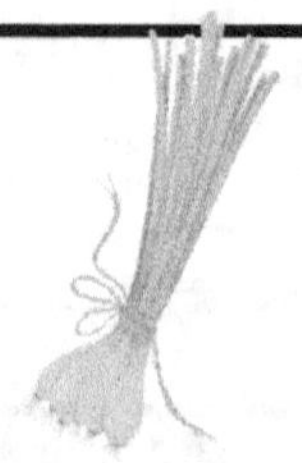

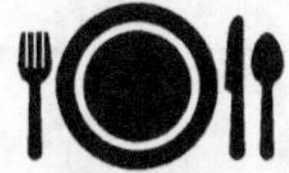 # Daily Healthy Eating Habits 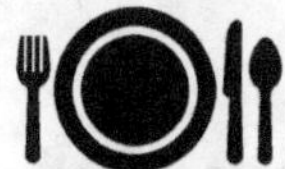

	Morning or Breakfast	Mid Day Or Lunch	Late Afternoon or Dinner	Evening Or Snacks
WATER- Drink 8-10 glasses or 3 L through out the day	⬡ ⬡ ⬡ ⬡ ⬡ ⬡ ⬡ ⬡			
Veggies & Fruits- try to eat 5 servings each day	🍎 🍎 🍎 🍎 🍎 🍎 🍎			
Protein- Eat a palm size at each meal				
Healthy Fats- Eat fingertip - thumb size at each meal				
Follow Hand Portion Sizes at each meal				
Listen to Hunger & Fullness Cues				
Eat Mindfully & Slowly- Follow the 20 min meal				
Stop eating starchy carbs at 7pm				
Followed the 80/20 or 90/10 rule				
Any skipped meals				

Daily Exercise Plan

Activity	Length of W/O	Weight	Reps	Sets	Speed	Distance	Calories Burned

My Daily Reflections

Date:

Top 3 Daily Goals

- [ ] _______________________
- [ ] _______________________
- [ ] _______________________

My Action Steps To Help Me Reach My Daily Goals Are:

My Top 3 Strengths Are

- [ ] _______________________
- [ ] _______________________
- [ ] _______________________

Today I Found Happiness In

3 Things I Love About My Body

- [ ] _______________________
- [ ] _______________________
- [ ] _______________________

I Am Grateful For

Daily Meal Planner

MEAL PLAN		Macros Counts
Breakfast		Calories______ Carbs:______ Protein:______ Fats:______
Mid Morning		Calories______ Carbs:______ Protein:______ Fats:______
Lunch		Calories______ Carbs:______ Protein:______ Fats:______
Afternoon		Calories______ Carbs:______ Protein:______ Fats:______
Dinner		Calories______ Carbs:______ Protein:______ Fats:______

	Calories	Carbs	Protein	Fats
Calculated Macros				
Daily Totals				

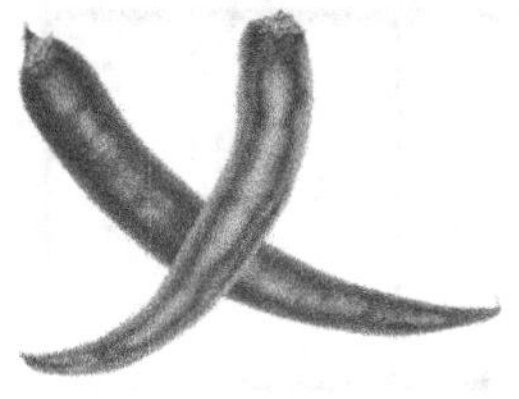
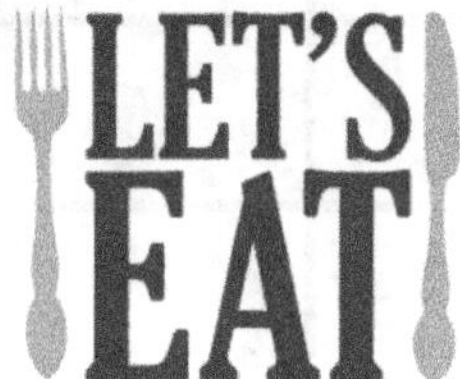

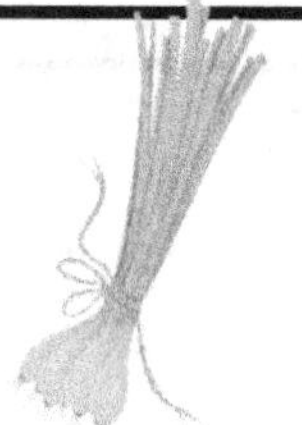

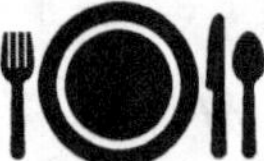 # Daily Healthy Eating Habits 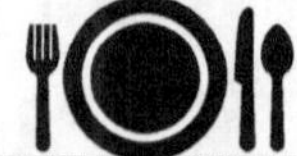

	Morning or Breakfast	Mid Day Or Lunch	Late Afternoon or Dinner	Evening Or Snacks
WATER- Drink 8-10 glasses or 3 L through out the day				
Veggies & Fruits- try to eat 5 servings each day				
Protein- Eat a palm size at each meal				
Healthy Fats- Eat fingertip - thumb size at each meal				
Follow Hand Portion Sizes at each meal				
Listen to Hunger & Fullness Cues				
Eat Mindfully & Slowly- Follow the 20 min meal				
Stop eating starchy carbs at 7pm				
Followed the 80/20 or 90/10 rule				
Any skipped meals				

Daily Exercise Plan

Activity	Length of W/O	Weight	Reps	Sets	Speed	Distance	Calories Burned

<table>
<tr><td>Week Of:</td><td></td><td colspan="2">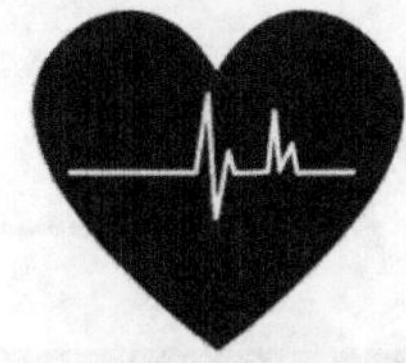</td><td colspan="2">Track Your Blood Sugar</td></tr>
</table>

Date	Wake Up	Pre-Lunch	Afternoon	Pre-Dinner	Bedtime

Results					
High					
Good					
Low					

Note Any Changes

WEEK 8 FROM: _______________

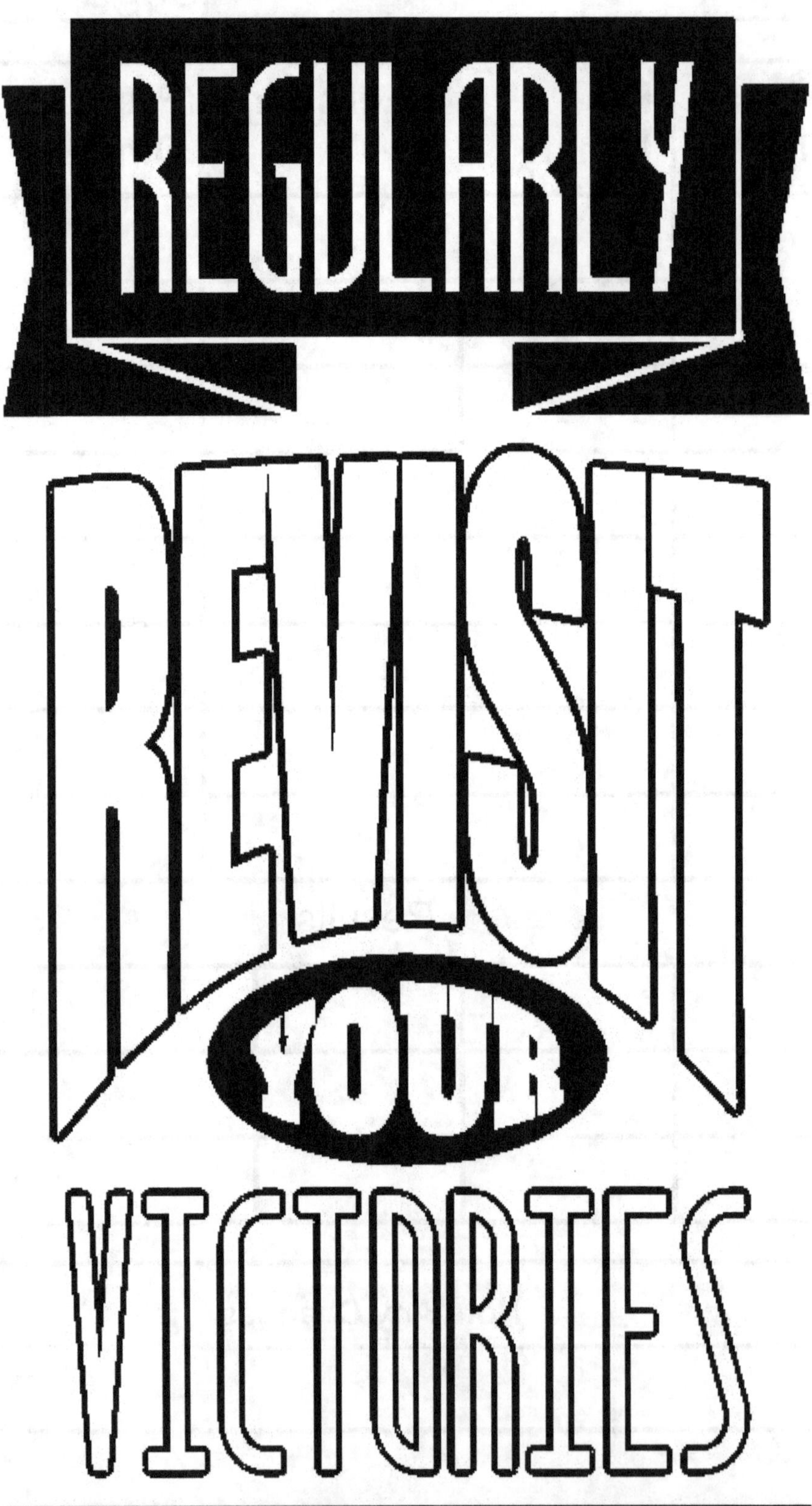

FACING FEAR

My Daily Reflections

Date:

★ Top 3 Daily Goals ★

- ☐ _______________________
- ☐ _______________________
- ☐ _______________________

My Action Steps To Help Me Reach My Daily Goals Are:

♥ My Top 3 Strengths Are ♥

- ☐ _______________________
- ☐ _______________________
- ☐ _______________________

Today I Found Happiness In

3 Things I Love About My Body

- ☐ _______________________
- ☐ _______________________
- ☐ _______________________

I Am Grateful For

Daily Meal Planner

MEAL PLAN		Macros Counts
Breakfast		Calories________ Carbs:________ Protein:________ Fats:________
Mid Morning		Calories________ Carbs:________ Protein:________ Fats:________
Lunch		Calories________ Carbs:________ Protein:________ Fats:________
Afternoon		Calories________ Carbs:________ Protein:________ Fats:________
Dinner		Calories________ Carbs:________ Protein:________ Fats:________

	Calories	Carbs	Protein	Fats
Calculated Macros				
Daily Totals				

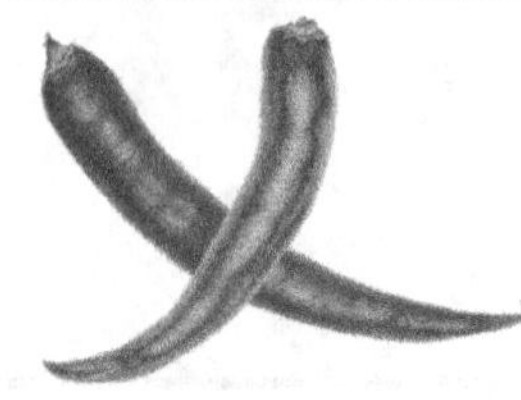
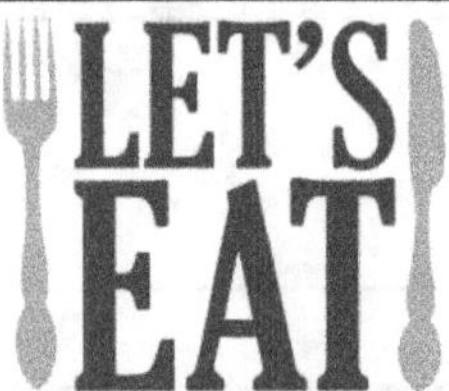

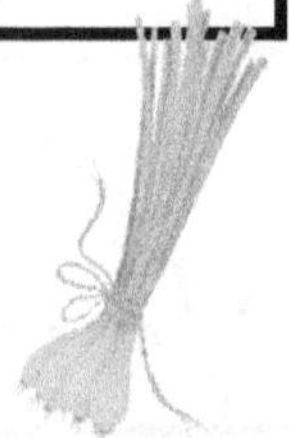

Daily Healthy Eating Habits

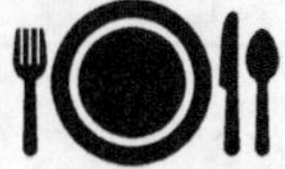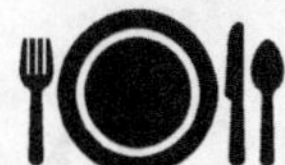

	Morning or Breakfast	Mid Day Or Lunch	Late Afternoon or Dinner	Evening Or Snacks
WATER- Drink 8-10 glasses or 3 L through out the day				
Veggies & Fruits- try to eat 5 servings each day				
Protein- Eat a palm size at each meal				
Healthy Fats- Eat fingertip - thumb size at each meal				
Follow Hand Portion Sizes at each meal				
Listen to Hunger & Fullness Cues				
Eat Mindfully & Slowly- Follow the 20 min meal				
Stop eating starchy carbs at 7pm				
Followed the 80/20 or 90/10 rule				
Any skipped meals				

Daily Exercise Plan

Activity	Length of W/O	Weight	Reps	Sets	Speed	Distance	Calories Burned

My Daily Reflections

Date:

⭐ Top 3 Daily Goals ⭐

My Action Steps To Help Me Reach My Daily Goals Are:

☐ ______________________________

☐ ______________________________

☐ ______________________________

♥ My Top 3 Strengths Are ♥

Today I Found Happiness In

☐ ______________________________

☐ ______________________________

☐ ______________________________

3 Things I Love About My Body

I Am Grateful For

☐ ______________________________

☐ ______________________________

☐ ______________________________

Daily Meal Planner

MEAL PLAN		Macros Counts
Breakfast		Calories________ Carbs:________ Protein:______ Fats:__________
Mid Morning		Calories________ Carbs:________ Protein:______ Fats:__________
Lunch		Calories________ Carbs:________ Protein:______ Fats:__________
Afternoon		Calories________ Carbs:________ Protein:______ Fats:__________
Dinner		Calories________ Carbs:________ Protein:______ Fats:__________

	Calories	Carbs	Protein	Fats
Calculated Macros				
Daily Totals				

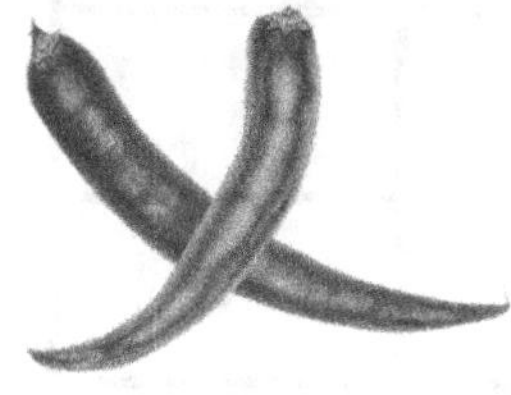

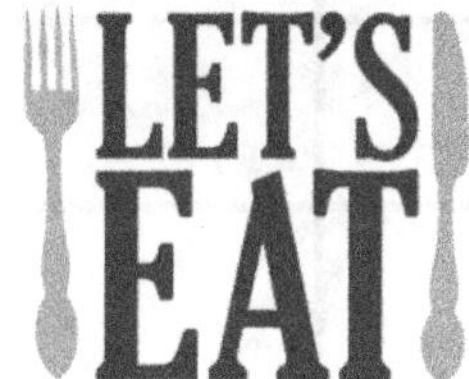

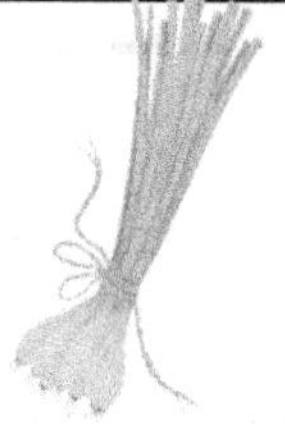

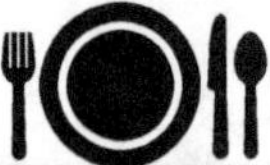 # Daily Healthy Eating Habits 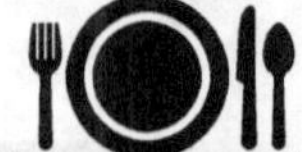

	Morning or Breakfast	Mid Day Or Lunch	Late Afternoon or Dinner	Evening Or Snacks
WATER- Drink 8-10 glasses or 3 L through out the day				
Veggies & Fruits- try to eat 5 servings each day				
Protein- Eat a palm size at each meal				
Healthy Fats- Eat fingertip - thumb size at each meal				
Follow Hand Portion Sizes at each meal				
Listen to Hunger & Fullness Cues				
Eat Mindfully & Slowly- Follow the 20 min meal				
Stop eating starchy carbs at 7pm				
Followed the 80/20 or 90/10 rule				
Any skipped meals				

Daily Exercise Plan

Activity	Length of W/O	Weight	Reps	Sets	Speed	Distance	Calories Burned

My Daily Reflections

Date:

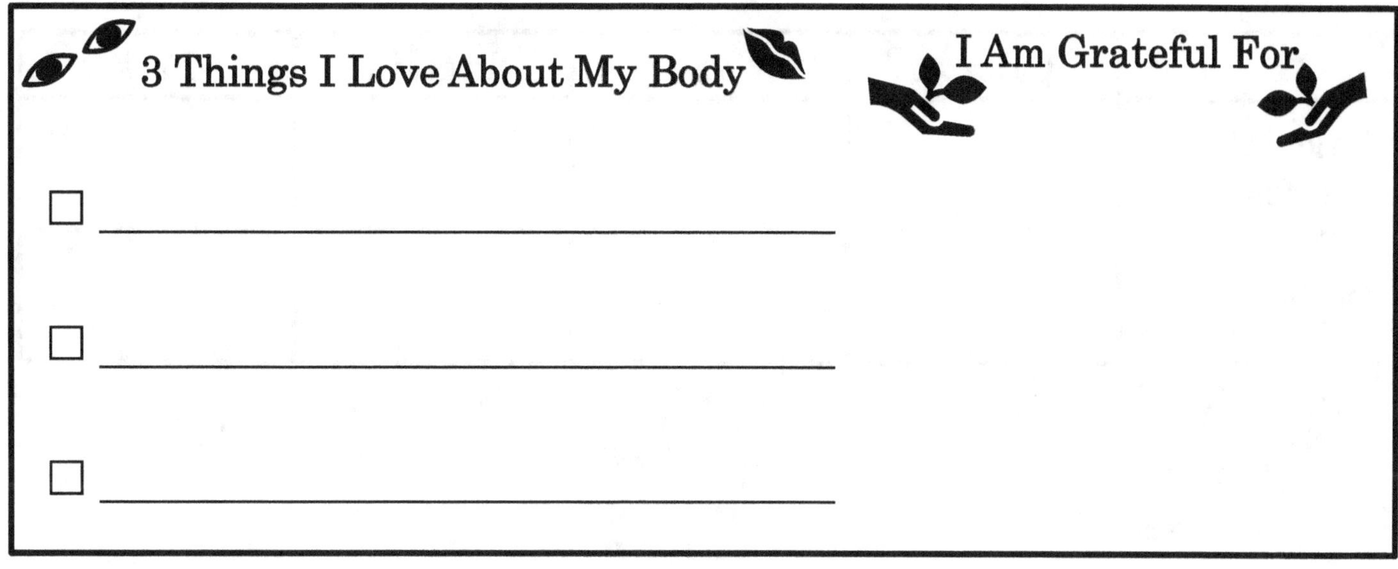

★ Top 3 Daily Goals ★

My Action Steps To Help Me
Reach My Daily Goals Are:

☐ _______________________

☐ _______________________

☐ _______________________

♥ My Top 3 Strengths Are ♥

Today I Found Happiness In

☐ _______________________

☐ _______________________

☐ _______________________

3 Things I Love About My Body

I Am Grateful For

☐ _______________________

☐ _______________________

☐ _______________________

Daily Meal Planner

MEAL PLAN		Macros Counts
Breakfast		Calories________ Carbs:________ Protein:________ Fats:__________
Mid Morning		Calories________ Carbs:________ Protein:________ Fats:__________
Lunch		Calories________ Carbs:________ Protein:________ Fats:__________
Afternoon		Calories________ Carbs:________ Protein:________ Fats:__________
Dinner		Calories________ Carbs:________ Protein:________ Fats:__________

	Calories	Carbs	Protein	Fats
Calculated Macros				
Daily Totals				

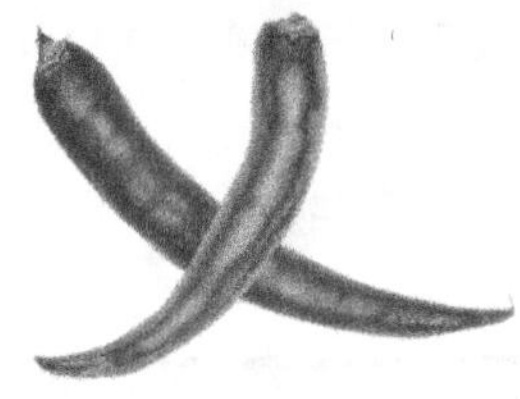
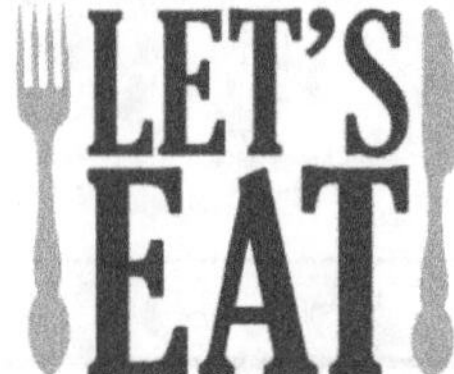

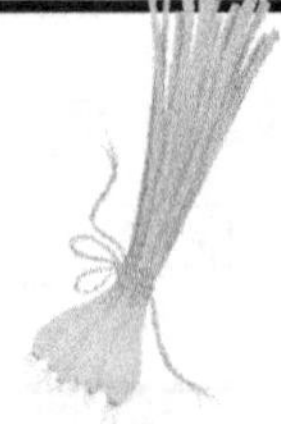

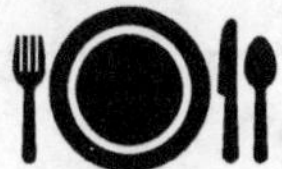 Daily Healthy Eating Habits 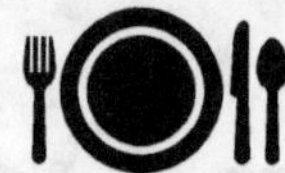

	Morning or Breakfast	Mid Day Or Lunch	Late Afternoon or Dinner	Evening Or Snacks
WATER- Drink 8-10 glasses or 3 L through out the day				
Veggies & Fruits- try to eat 5 servings each day				
Protein- Eat a palm size at each meal				
Healthy Fats- Eat fingertip - thumb size at each meal				
Follow Hand Portion Sizes at each meal				
Listen to Hunger & Fullness Cues				
Eat Mindfully & Slowly- Follow the 20 min meal				
Stop eating starchy carbs at 7pm				
Followed the 80/20 or 90/10 rule				
Any skipped meals				

Daily Exercise Plan

Activity	Length of W/O	Weight	Reps	Sets	Speed	Distance	Calories Burned

My Daily Reflections

Date:

★ Top 3 Daily Goals ★

My Action Steps To Help Me Reach My Daily Goals Are:

- ☐ _______________________
- ☐ _______________________
- ☐ _______________________

♥ My Top 3 Strengths Are ♥

Today I Found Happiness In

- ☐ _______________________
- ☐ _______________________
- ☐ _______________________

---

3 Things I Love About My Body

I Am Grateful For

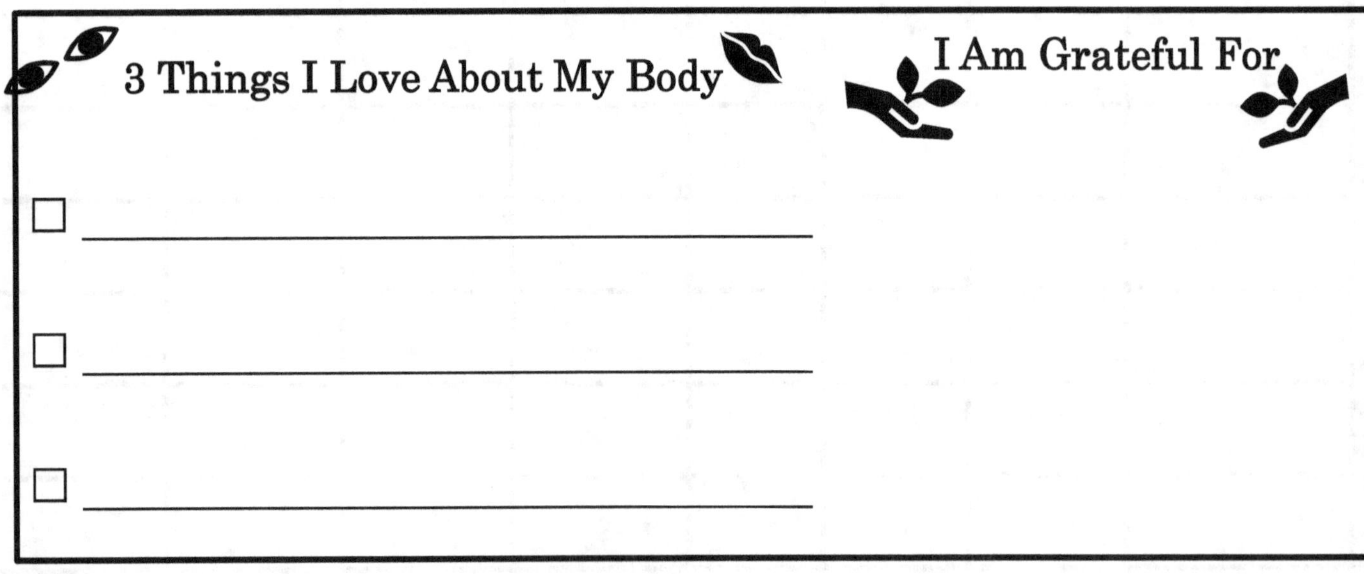

- ☐ _______________________
- ☐ _______________________
- ☐ _______________________

Daily Meal Planner

MEAL PLAN		Macros Counts
Breakfast		Calories______ Carbs:______ Protein:______ Fats:______
Mid Morning		Calories______ Carbs:______ Protein:______ Fats:______
Lunch		Calories______ Carbs:______ Protein:______ Fats:______
Afternoon		Calories______ Carbs:______ Protein:______ Fats:______
Dinner		Calories______ Carbs:______ Protein:______ Fats:______

	Calories	Carbs	Protein	Fats
Calculated Macros				
Daily Totals				

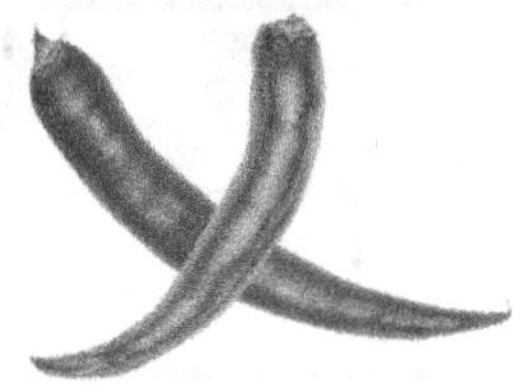

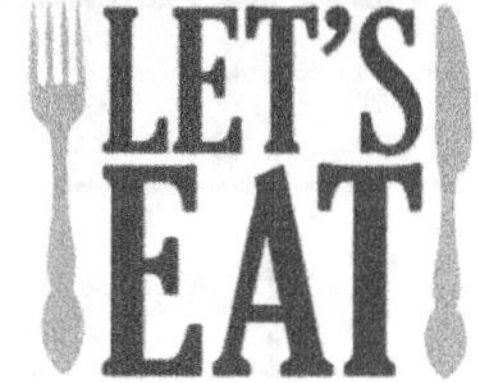

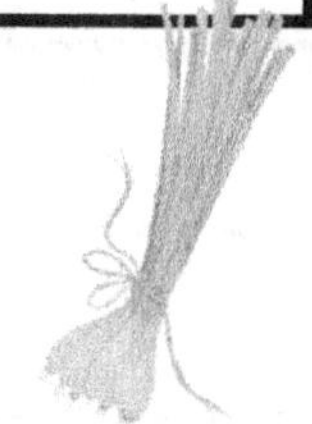

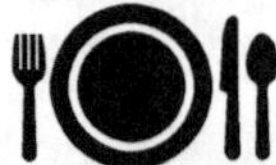 # Daily Healthy Eating Habits 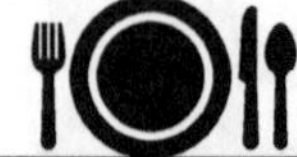

	Morning or Breakfast	Mid Day Or Lunch	Late Afternoon or Dinner	Evening Or Snacks
WATER- Drink 8-10 glasses or 3 L through out the day				
Veggies & Fruits- try to eat 5 servings each day				
Protein- Eat a palm size at each meal				
Healthy Fats- Eat fingertip - thumb size at each meal				
Follow Hand Portion Sizes at each meal				
Listen to Hunger & Fullness Cues				
Eat Mindfully & Slowly- Follow the 20 min meal				
Stop eating starchy carbs at 7pm				
Followed the 80/20 or 90/10 rule				
Any skipped meals				

Daily Exercise Plan

Activity	Length of W/O	Weight	Reps	Sets	Speed	Distance	Calories Burned

My Daily Reflections

Date:

Top 3 Daily Goals

My Action Steps To Help Me Reach My Daily Goals Are:

My Top 3 Strengths Are

Today I Found Happiness In

3 Things I Love About My Body

I Am Grateful For

Daily Meal Planner

MEAL PLAN		Macros Counts
Breakfast		Calories______ Carbs:______ Protein:______ Fats:______
Mid Morning		Calories______ Carbs:______ Protein:______ Fats:______
Lunch		Calories______ Carbs:______ Protein:______ Fats:______
Afternoon		Calories______ Carbs:______ Protein:______ Fats:______
Dinner		Calories______ Carbs:______ Protein:______ Fats:______

	Calories	Carbs	Protein	Fats
Calculated Macros				
Daily Totals				

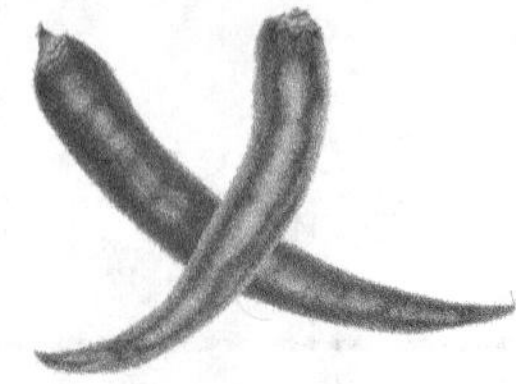

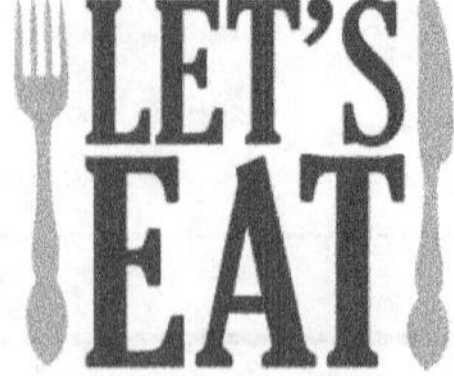

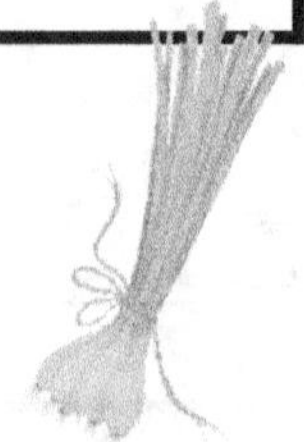

Daily Healthy Eating Habits

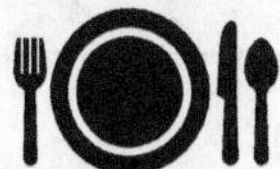 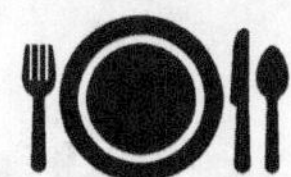

	Morning or Breakfast	Mid Day Or Lunch	Late Afternoon or Dinner	Evening Or Snacks
WATER- Drink 8-10 glasses or 3 L through out the day				
Veggies & Fruits- try to eat 5 servings each day				
Protein- Eat a palm size at each meal				
Healthy Fats- Eat fingertip - thumb size at each meal				
Follow Hand Portion Sizes at each meal				
Listen to Hunger & Fullness Cues				
Eat Mindfully & Slowly- Follow the 20 min meal				
Stop eating starchy carbs at 7pm				
Followed the 80/20 or 90/10 rule				
Any skipped meals				

Daily Exercise Plan

Activity	Length of W/O	Weight	Reps	Sets	Speed	Distance	Calories Burned

My Daily Reflections

Date:

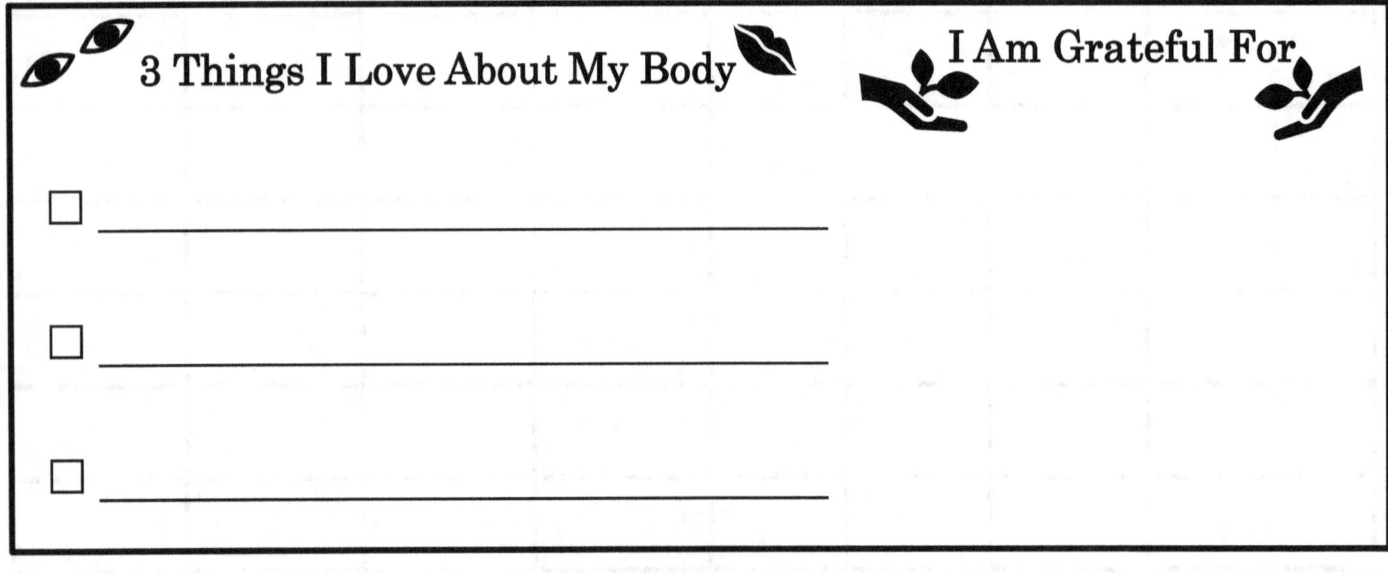

★ Top 3 Daily Goals ★

- ☐ ___________________________
- ☐ ___________________________
- ☐ ___________________________

My Action Steps To Help Me Reach My Daily Goals Are:

♥ My Top 3 Strengths Are ♥

- ☐ ___________________________
- ☐ ___________________________
- ☐ ___________________________

Today I Found Happiness In

3 Things I Love About My Body

- ☐ ___________________________
- ☐ ___________________________
- ☐ ___________________________

I Am Grateful For

Daily Meal Planner

	MEAL PLAN	Macros Counts
Breakfast		Calories_______ Carbs:_______ Protein:______ Fats:_________
Mid Morning		Calories_______ Carbs:_______ Protein:______ Fats:_________
Lunch		Calories_______ Carbs:_______ Protein:______ Fats:_________
Afternoon		Calories_______ Carbs:_______ Protein:______ Fats:_________
Dinner		Calories_______ Carbs:_______ Protein:______ Fats:_________

	Calories	Carbs	Protein	Fats
Calculated Macros				
Daily Totals				

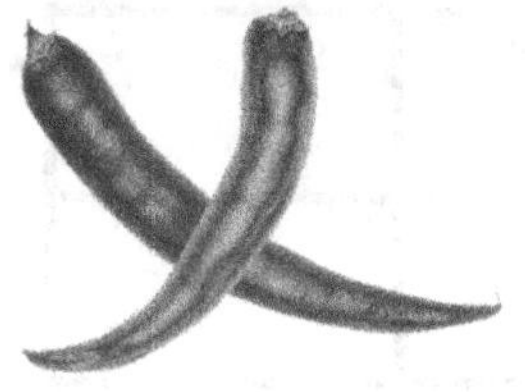

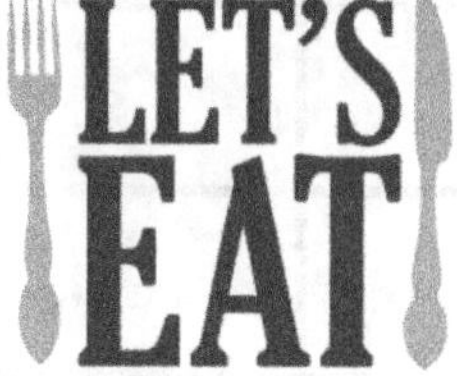

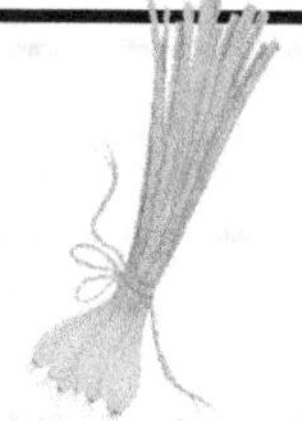

Daily Healthy Eating Habits

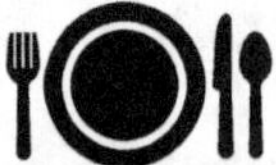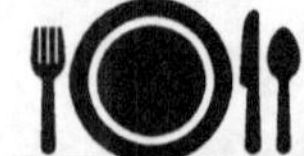

	Morning or Breakfast	Mid Day Or Lunch	Late Afternoon or Dinner	Evening Or Snacks
WATER- Drink 8-10 glasses or 3 L through out the day				
Veggies & Fruits- try to eat 5 servings each day				
Protein- Eat a palm size at each meal				
Healthy Fats- Eat fingertip - thumb size at each meal				
Follow Hand Portion Sizes at each meal				
Listen to Hunger & Fullness Cues				
Eat Mindfully & Slowly- Follow the 20 min meal				
Stop eating starchy carbs at 7pm				
Followed the 80/20 or 90/10 rule				
Any skipped meals				

Daily Exercise Plan

Activity	Length of W/O	Weight	Reps	Sets	Speed	Distance	Calories Burned

My Daily Reflections

Date:

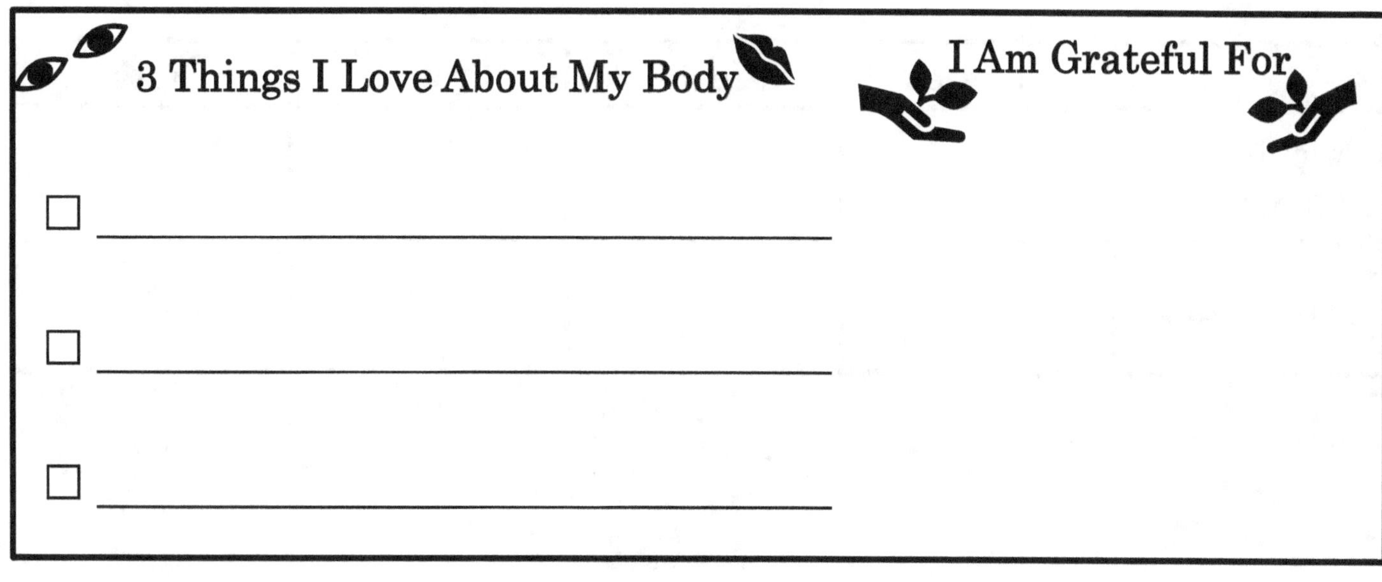

Top 3 Daily Goals

- ☐ ________________________
- ☐ ________________________
- ☐ ________________________

My Action Steps To Help Me Reach My Daily Goals Are:

My Top 3 Strengths Are

- ☐ ________________________
- ☐ ________________________
- ☐ ________________________

Today I Found Happiness In

3 Things I Love About My Body

- ☐ ________________________
- ☐ ________________________
- ☐ ________________________

I Am Grateful For

Daily Meal Planner

MEAL PLAN		Macros Counts
Breakfast		Calories________ Carbs:________ Protein:________ Fats:________
Mid Morning		Calories________ Carbs:________ Protein:________ Fats:________
Lunch		Calories________ Carbs:________ Protein:________ Fats:________
Afternoon		Calories________ Carbs:________ Protein:________ Fats:________
Dinner		Calories________ Carbs:________ Protein:________ Fats:________

	Calories	Carbs	Protein	Fats
Calculated Macros				
Daily Totals				

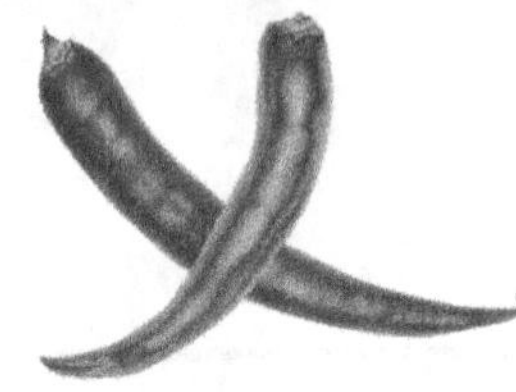
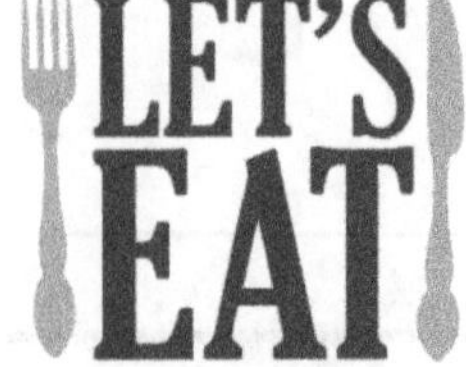

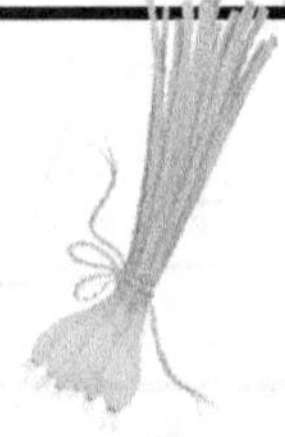

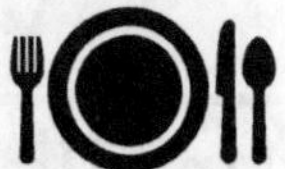 # Daily Healthy Eating Habits 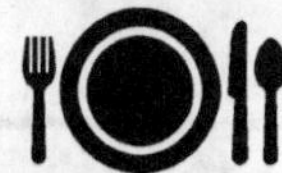

	Morning or Breakfast	Mid Day Or Lunch	Late Afternoon or Dinner	Evening Or Snacks
WATER- Drink 8-10 glasses or 3 L through out the day				
Veggies & Fruits- try to eat 5 servings each day				
Protein- Eat a palm size at each meal				
Healthy Fats- Eat fingertip - thumb size at each meal				
Follow Hand Portion Sizes at each meal				
Listen to Hunger & Fullness Cues				
Eat Mindfully & Slowly- Follow the 20 min meal				
Stop eating starchy carbs at 7pm				
Followed the 80/20 or 90/10 rule				
Any skipped meals				

Daily Exercise Plan

Activity	Length of W/O	Weight	Reps	Sets	Speed	Distance	Calories Burned

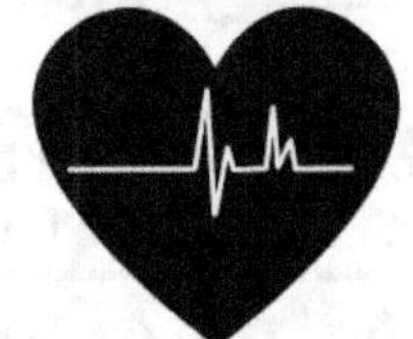

Track Your Blood Sugar

Date	Wake Up	Pre-Lunch	Afternoon	Pre-Dinner	Bedtime

Results

High				
Good				
Low				

Note Any Changes

WEEK 9 FROM: ___________

REWARD Yourself FOR STICKING TO NEW HABITS

My Daily Reflections

Date:

★ Top 3 Daily Goals ★

My Action Steps To Help Me
Reach My Daily Goals Are:

- [ ] _______________________
- [ ] _______________________
- [ ] _______________________

♥ My Top 3 Strengths Are ♥

Today I Found Happiness In

- [ ] _______________________
- [ ] _______________________
- [ ] _______________________

3 Things I Love About My Body

I Am Grateful For

- [ ] _______________________
- [ ] _______________________
- [ ] _______________________

Daily Meal Planner

MEAL PLAN		Macros Counts
Breakfast		Calories______ Carbs:______ Protein:______ Fats:________
Mid Morning		Calories______ Carbs:______ Protein:______ Fats:________
Lunch		Calories______ Carbs:______ Protein:______ Fats:________
Afternoon		Calories______ Carbs:______ Protein:______ Fats:________
Dinner		Calories______ Carbs:______ Protein:______ Fats:________

	Calories	Carbs	Protein	Fats
Calculated Macros				
Daily Totals				

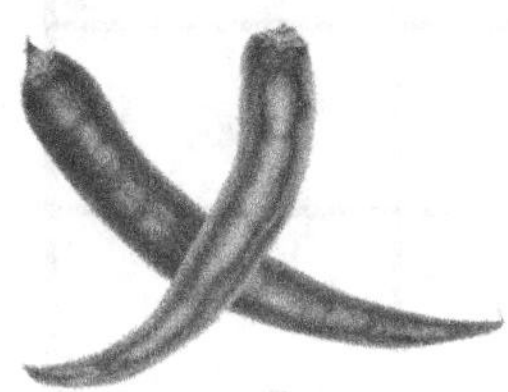
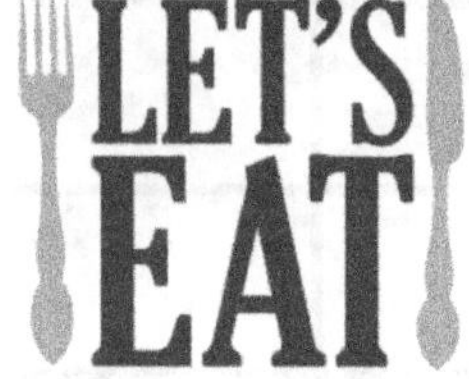

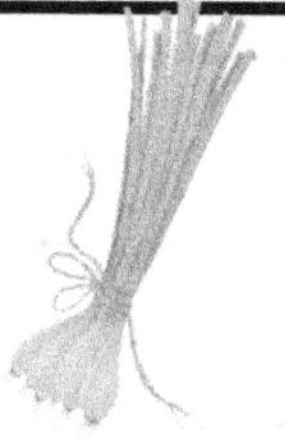

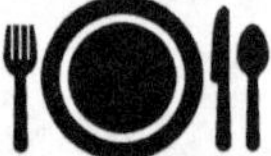 # Daily Healthy Eating Habits 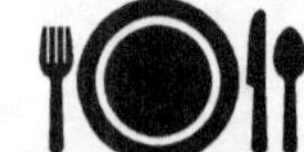

	Morning or Breakfast	Mid Day Or Lunch	Late Afternoon or Dinner	Evening Or Snacks
WATER- Drink 8-10 glasses or 3 L through out the day				
Veggies & Fruits- try to eat 5 servings each day				
Protein- Eat a palm size at each meal				
Healthy Fats- Eat fingertip - thumb size at each meal				
Follow Hand Portion Sizes at each meal				
Listen to Hunger & Fullness Cues				
Eat Mindfully & Slowly- Follow the 20 min meal				
Stop eating starchy carbs at 7pm				
Followed the 80/20 or 90/10 rule				
Any skipped meals				

Daily Exercise Plan

Activity	Length of W/O	Weight	Reps	Sets	Speed	Distance	Calories Burned

My Daily Reflections

Date:

Top 3 Daily Goals

- [ ] _______________________
- [ ] _______________________
- [ ] _______________________

My Action Steps To Help Me Reach My Daily Goals Are:

My Top 3 Strengths Are

- [ ] _______________________
- [ ] _______________________
- [ ] _______________________

Today I Found Happiness In

3 Things I Love About My Body

- [ ] _______________________
- [ ] _______________________
- [ ] _______________________

I Am Grateful For

Daily Meal Planner

MEAL PLAN		Macros Counts
Breakfast		Calories________ Carbs:________ Protein:______ Fats:__________
Mid Morning		Calories________ Carbs:________ Protein:______ Fats:__________
Lunch		Calories________ Carbs:________ Protein:______ Fats:__________
Afternoon		Calories________ Carbs:________ Protein:______ Fats:__________
Dinner		Calories________ Carbs:________ Protein:______ Fats:__________

	Calories	Carbs	Protein	Fats
Calculated Macros				
Daily Totals				

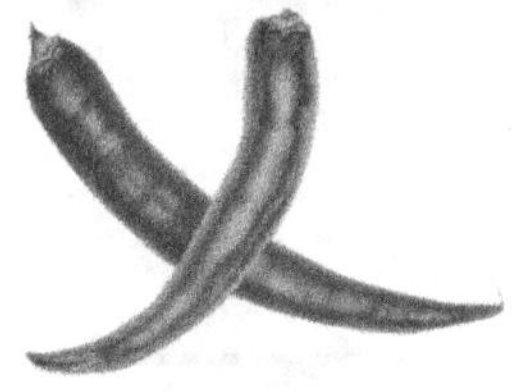

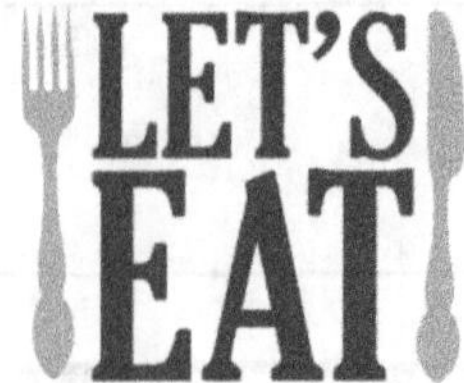

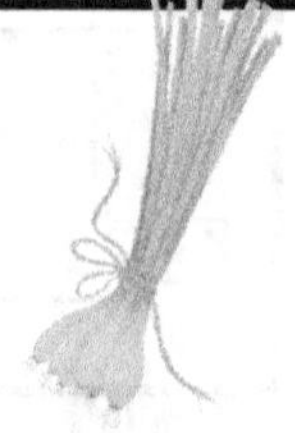

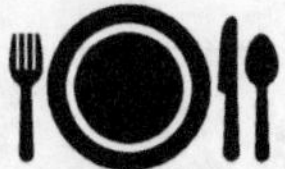 # Daily Healthy Eating Habits 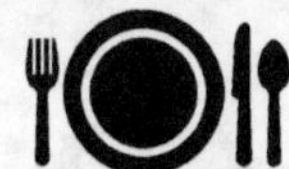

	Morning or Breakfast	Mid Day Or Lunch	Late Afternoon or Dinner	Evening Or Snacks
WATER- Drink 8-10 glasses or 3 L through out the day	◊ ◊ ◊ ◊ ◊ ◊ ◊			
Veggies & Fruits- try to eat 5 servings each day	🍎 🍎 🍎 🍎 🍎 🍎 🍎			
Protein- Eat a palm size at each meal				
Healthy Fats- Eat fingertip - thumb size at each meal				
Follow Hand Portion Sizes at each meal				
Listen to Hunger & Fullness Cues				
Eat Mindfully & Slowly- Follow the 20 min meal				
Stop eating starchy carbs at 7pm				
Followed the 80/20 or 90/10 rule				
Any skipped meals				

Daily Exercise Plan

Activity	Length of W/O	Weight	Reps	Sets	Speed	Distance	Calories Burned

My Daily Reflections

Date:

Top 3 Daily Goals

- ☐ ___________________
- ☐ ___________________
- ☐ ___________________

My Action Steps To Help Me Reach My Daily Goals Are:

My Top 3 Strengths Are

- ☐ ___________________
- ☐ ___________________
- ☐ ___________________

Today I Found Happiness In

3 Things I Love About My Body

- ☐ ___________________
- ☐ ___________________
- ☐ ___________________

I Am Grateful For

Daily Meal Planner

MEAL PLAN		Macros Counts
Breakfast		Calories______ Carbs:_______ Protein:______ Fats:________
Mid Morning		Calories______ Carbs:_______ Protein:______ Fats:________
Lunch		Calories______ Carbs:_______ Protein:______ Fats:________
Afternoon		Calories______ Carbs:_______ Protein:______ Fats:________
Dinner		Calories______ Carbs:_______ Protein:______ Fats:________

	Calories	Carbs	Protein	Fats
Calculated Macros				
Daily Totals				

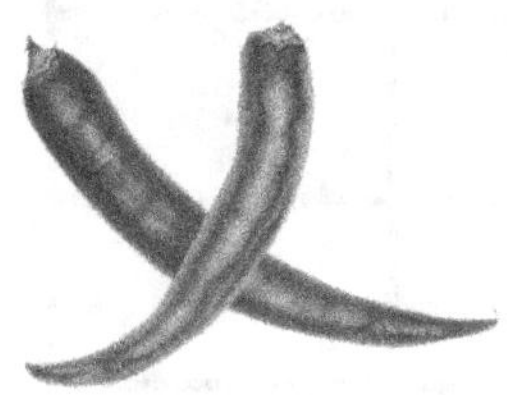
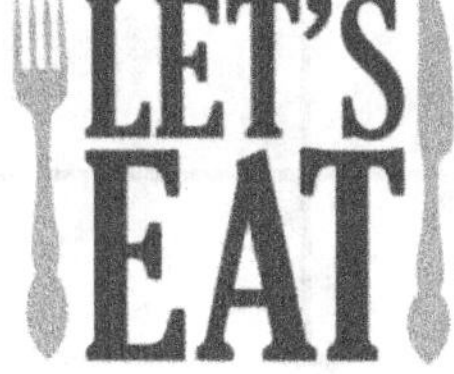

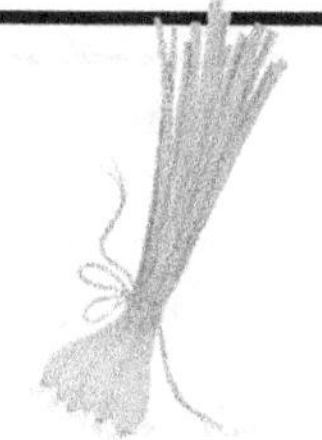

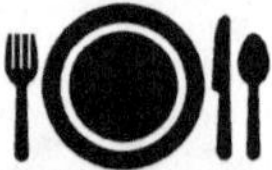 Daily Healthy Eating Habits 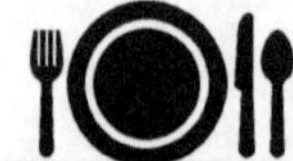

	Morning or Breakfast	Mid Day Or Lunch	Late Afternoon or Dinner	Evening Or Snacks
WATER- Drink 8-10 glasses or 3 L through out the day				
Veggies & Fruits- try to eat 5 servings each day				
Protein- Eat a palm size at each meal				
Healthy Fats- Eat fingertip - thumb size at each meal				
Follow Hand Portion Sizes at each meal				
Listen to Hunger & Fullness Cues				
Eat Mindfully & Slowly- Follow the 20 min meal				
Stop eating starchy carbs at 7pm				
Followed the 80/20 or 90/10 rule				
Any skipped meals				

Daily Exercise Plan

Activity	Length of W/O	Weight	Reps	Sets	Speed	Distance	Calories Burned

My Daily Reflections

Date:

Top 3 Daily Goals

- ☐ _______________________
- ☐ _______________________
- ☐ _______________________

My Action Steps To Help Me Reach My Daily Goals Are:

My Top 3 Strengths Are

- ☐ _______________________
- ☐ _______________________
- ☐ _______________________

Today I Found Happiness In

3 Things I Love About My Body

- ☐ _______________________
- ☐ _______________________
- ☐ _______________________

I Am Grateful For

Daily Meal Planner

MEAL PLAN		Macros Counts
Breakfast		Calories________ Carbs:________ Protein:________ Fats:__________
Mid Morning		Calories________ Carbs:________ Protein:________ Fats:__________
Lunch		Calories________ Carbs:________ Protein:________ Fats:__________
Afternoon		Calories________ Carbs:________ Protein:________ Fats:__________
Dinner		Calories________ Carbs:________ Protein:________ Fats:__________

	Calories	Carbs	Protein	Fats
Calculated Macros				
Daily Totals				

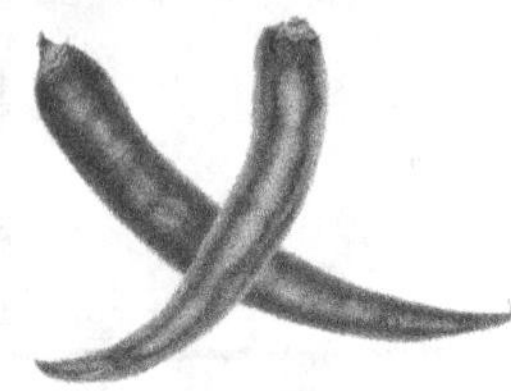
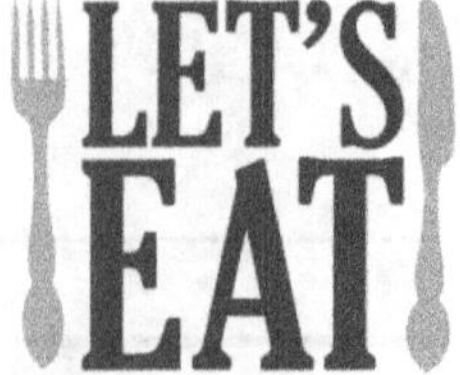

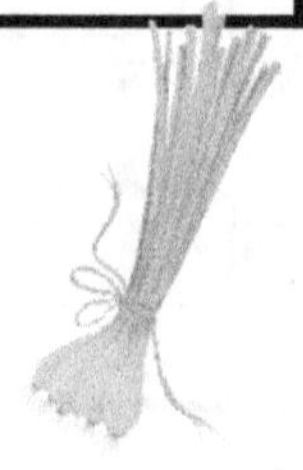

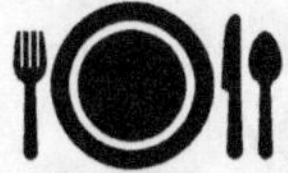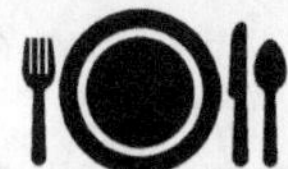

Daily Healthy Eating Habits

	Morning or Breakfast	Mid Day Or Lunch	Late Afternoon or Dinner	Evening Or Snacks
WATER- Drink 8-10 glasses or 3 L through out the day				
Veggies & Fruits- try to eat 5 servings each day				
Protein- Eat a palm size at each meal				
Healthy Fats- Eat fingertip - thumb size at each meal				
Follow Hand Portion Sizes at each meal				
Listen to Hunger & Fullness Cues				
Eat Mindfully & Slowly- Follow the 20 min meal				
Stop eating starchy carbs at 7pm				
Followed the 80/20 or 90/10 rule				
Any skipped meals				

Daily Exercise Plan

Activity	Length of W/O	Weight	Reps	Sets	Speed	Distance	Calories Burned

My Daily Reflections

★ Top 3 Daily Goals ★

- ☐ ___________________________
- ☐ ___________________________
- ☐ ___________________________

My Action Steps To Help Me Reach My Daily Goals Are:

♥ My Top 3 Strengths Are ♥

- ☐ ___________________________
- ☐ ___________________________
- ☐ ___________________________

Today I Found Happiness In

3 Things I Love About My Body

- ☐ ___________________________
- ☐ ___________________________
- ☐ ___________________________

I Am Grateful For

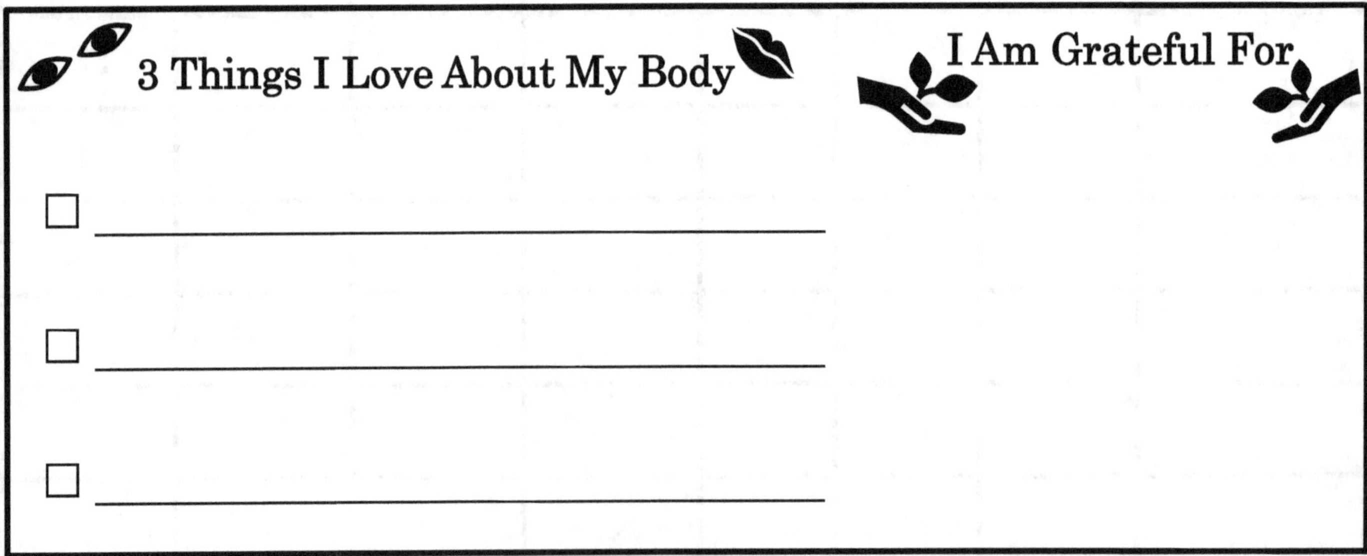

Daily Meal Planner

	MEAL PLAN	Macros Counts
Breakfast		Calories______ Carbs:_______ Protein:______ Fats:_________
Mid Morning		Calories______ Carbs:_______ Protein:______ Fats:_________
Lunch		Calories______ Carbs:_______ Protein:______ Fats:_________
Afternoon		Calories______ Carbs:_______ Protein:______ Fats:_________
Dinner		Calories______ Carbs:_______ Protein:______ Fats:_________

	Calories	Carbs	Protein	Fats
Calculated Macros				
Daily Totals				

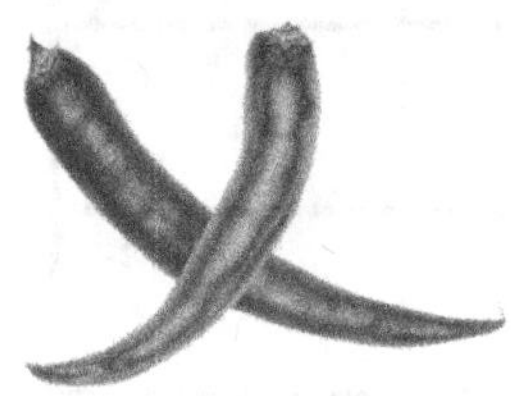
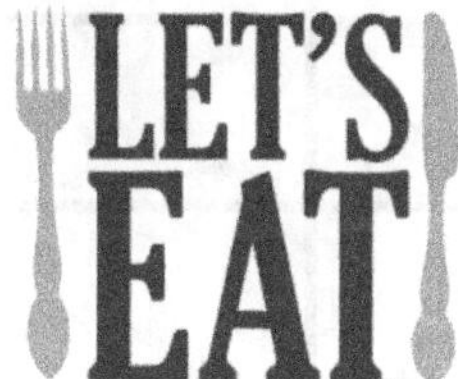

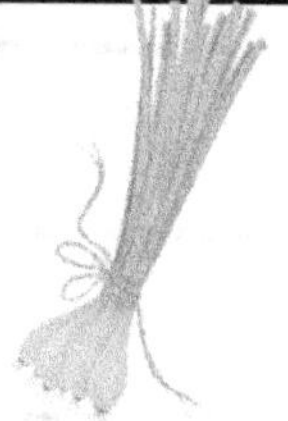

Daily Healthy Eating Habits

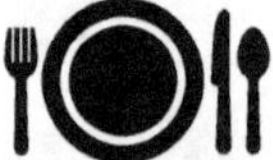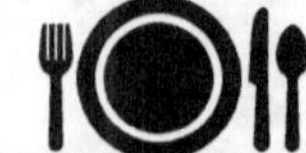

	Morning or Breakfast	Mid Day Or Lunch	Late Afternoon or Dinner	Evening Or Snacks
WATER- Drink 8-10 glasses or 3 L through out the day				
Veggies & Fruits- try to eat 5 servings each day				
Protein- Eat a palm size at each meal				
Healthy Fats- Eat fingertip - thumb size at each meal				
Follow Hand Portion Sizes at each meal				
Listen to Hunger & Fullness Cues				
Eat Mindfully & Slowly- Follow the 20 min meal				
Stop eating starchy carbs at 7pm				
Followed the 80/20 or 90/10 rule				
Any skipped meals				

Daily Exercise Plan

Activity	Length of W/O	Weight	Reps	Sets	Speed	Distance	Calories Burned

My Daily Reflections

Date:

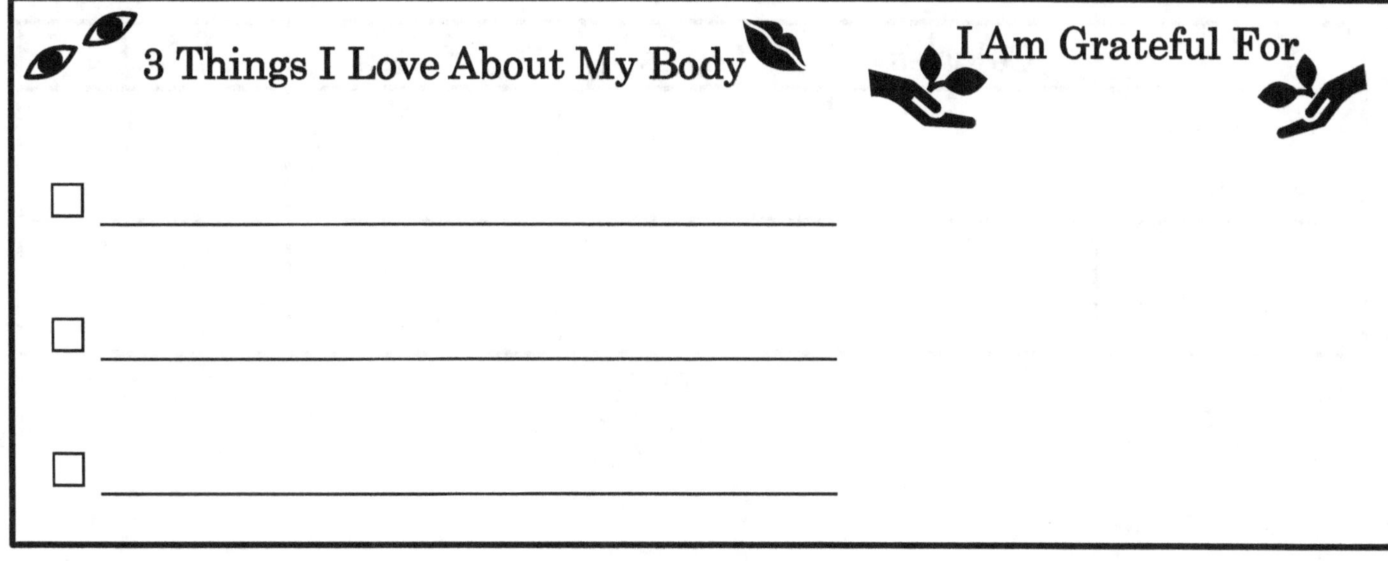

⭐ Top 3 Daily Goals ⭐

- ☐ _______________
- ☐ _______________
- ☐ _______________

My Action Steps To Help Me Reach My Daily Goals Are:

❤ My Top 3 Strengths Are ❤

- ☐ _______________
- ☐ _______________
- ☐ _______________

Today I Found Happiness In

3 Things I Love About My Body

- ☐ _______________
- ☐ _______________
- ☐ _______________

I Am Grateful For

Daily Meal Planner

MEAL PLAN		Macros Counts
Breakfast		Calories________ Carbs:________ Protein:_______ Fats:__________
Mid Morning		Calories________ Carbs:________ Protein:_______ Fats:__________
Lunch		Calories________ Carbs:________ Protein:_______ Fats:__________
Afternoon		Calories________ Carbs:________ Protein:_______ Fats:__________
Dinner		Calories________ Carbs:________ Protein:_______ Fats:__________

	Calories	Carbs	Protein	Fats
Calculated Macros				
Daily Totals				

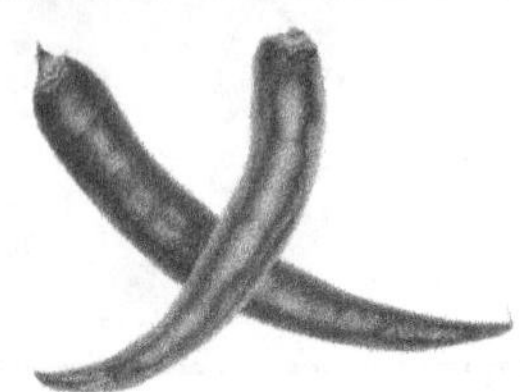
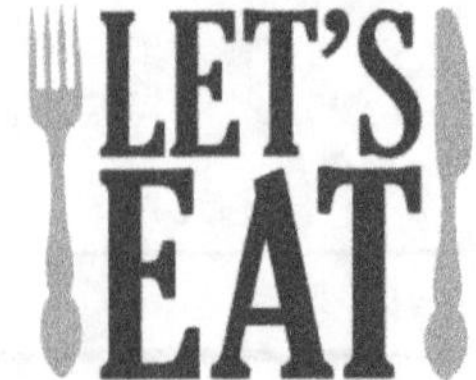

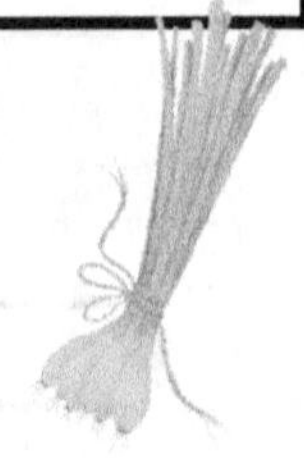

Daily Healthy Eating Habits

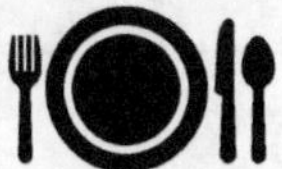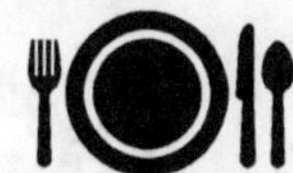

	Morning or Breakfast	Mid Day Or Lunch	Late Afternoon or Dinner	Evening Or Snacks
WATER- Drink 8-10 glasses or 3 L through out the day				
Veggies & Fruits- try to eat 5 servings each day				
Protein- Eat a palm size at each meal				
Healthy Fats- Eat fingertip - thumb size at each meal				
Follow Hand Portion Sizes at each meal				
Listen to Hunger & Fullness Cues				
Eat Mindfully & Slowly- Follow the 20 min meal				
Stop eating starchy carbs at 7pm				
Followed the 80/20 or 90/10 rule				
Any skipped meals				

Daily Exercise Plan

Activity	Length of W/O	Weight	Reps	Sets	Speed	Distance	Calories Burned

My Daily Reflections

Date:

★ Top 3 Daily Goals ★

- ☐ _______________________
- ☐ _______________________
- ☐ _______________________

My Action Steps To Help Me Reach My Daily Goals Are:

♥ My Top 3 Strengths Are ♥

- ☐ _______________________
- ☐ _______________________
- ☐ _______________________

Today I Found Happiness In

---

3 Things I Love About My Body

- ☐ _______________________
- ☐ _______________________
- ☐ _______________________

I Am Grateful For

Daily Meal Planner

MEAL PLAN		Macros Counts
Breakfast		Calories________ Carbs:________ Protein:______ Fats:_________
Mid Morning		Calories________ Carbs:________ Protein:______ Fats:_________
Lunch		Calories________ Carbs:________ Protein:______ Fats:_________
Afternoon		Calories________ Carbs:________ Protein:______ Fats:_________
Dinner		Calories________ Carbs:________ Protein:______ Fats:_________

	Calories	Carbs	Protein	Fats
Calculated Macros				
Daily Totals				

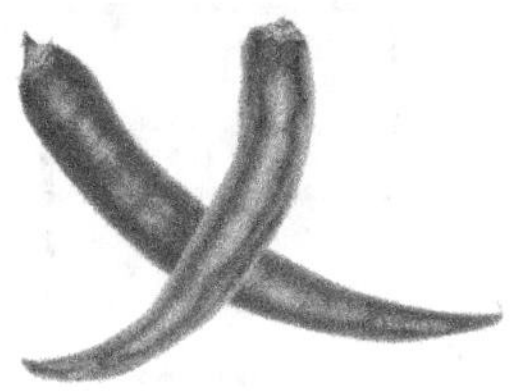
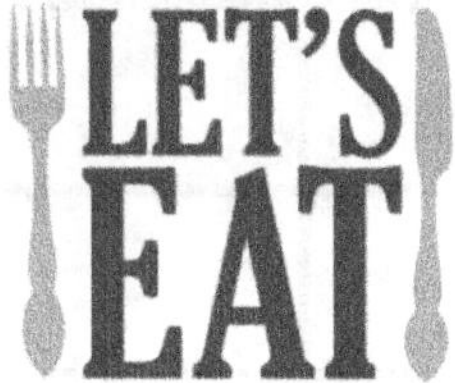

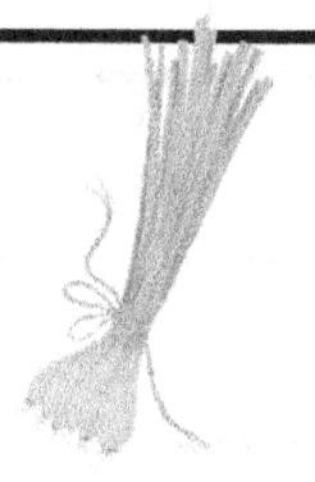

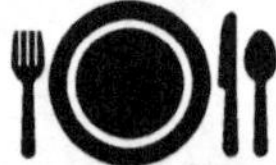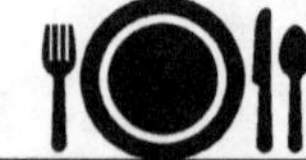

Daily Healthy Eating Habits

	Morning or Breakfast	Mid Day Or Lunch	Late Afternoon or Dinner	Evening Or Snacks
WATER- Drink 8-10 glasses or 3 L through out the day				
Veggies & Fruits- try to eat 5 servings each day				
Protein- Eat a palm size at each meal				
Healthy Fats- Eat fingertip - thumb size at each meal				
Follow Hand Portion Sizes at each meal				
Listen to Hunger & Fullness Cues				
Eat Mindfully & Slowly- Follow the 20 min meal				
Stop eating starchy carbs at 7pm				
Followed the 80/20 or 90/10 rule				
Any skipped meals				

Daily Exercise Plan

Activity	Length of W/O	Weight	Reps	Sets	Speed	Distance	Calories Burned

<table>
<tr><td>Week Of:</td><td colspan="4">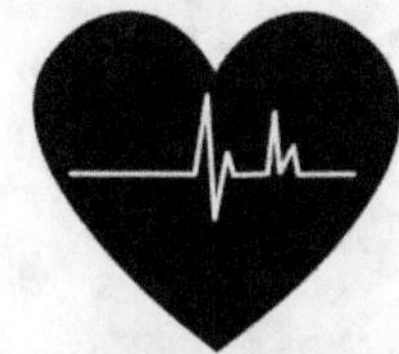</td><td colspan="1">Track Your Blood Sugar</td></tr>
</table>

Date	Wake Up	Pre-Lunch	Afternoon	Pre-Dinner	Bedtime

Results

High					
Good					
Low					

Note Any Changes

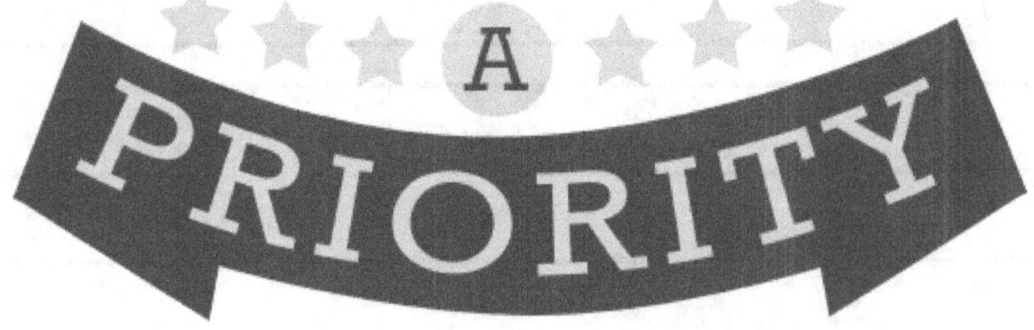

MAKE
YOUR
OWN
HAPPINESS
A
PRIORITY
LOOKING OUT FOR #1

My Daily Reflections

Date:

★ Top 3 Daily Goals ★

My Action Steps To Help Me
Reach My Daily Goals Are:

☐ __________________________

☐ __________________________

☐ __________________________

♥ My Top 3 Strengths Are ♥

Today I Found Happiness In

☐ __________________________

☐ __________________________

☐ __________________________

3 Things I Love About My Body

I Am Grateful For

☐ __________________________

☐ __________________________

☐ __________________________

Daily Meal Planner

MEAL PLAN		Macros Counts
Breakfast		Calories_______ Carbs:_______ Protein:______ Fats:_________
Mid Morning		Calories_______ Carbs:_______ Protein:______ Fats:_________
Lunch		Calories_______ Carbs:_______ Protein:______ Fats:_________
Afternoon		Calories_______ Carbs:_______ Protein:______ Fats:_________
Dinner		Calories_______ Carbs:_______ Protein:______ Fats:_________

	Calories	Carbs	Protein	Fats
Calculated Macros				
Daily Totals				

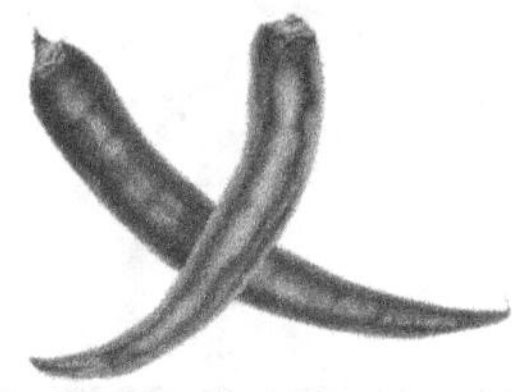
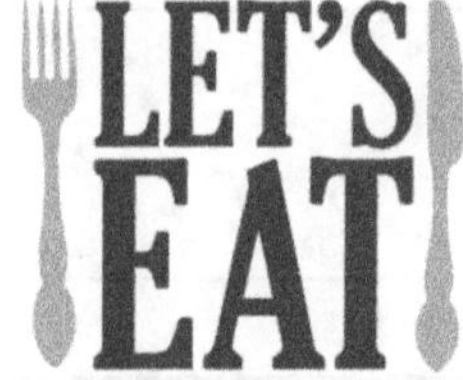

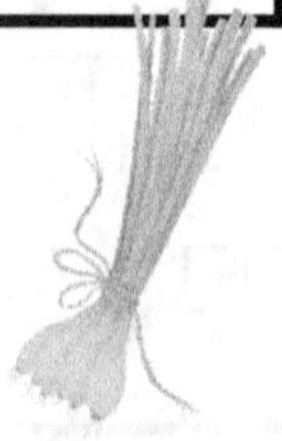

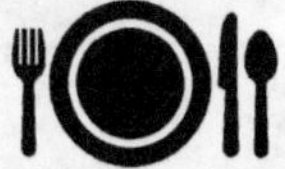 # Daily Healthy Eating Habits 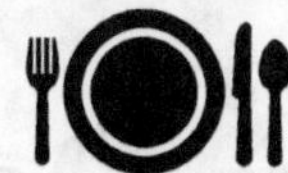

	Morning or Breakfast	Mid Day Or Lunch	Late Afternoon or Dinner	Evening Or Snacks
WATER- Drink 8-10 glasses or 3 L through out the day				
Veggies & Fruits- try to eat 5 servings each day				
Protein- Eat a palm size at each meal				
Healthy Fats- Eat fingertip - thumb size at each meal				
Follow Hand Portion Sizes at each meal				
Listen to Hunger & Fullness Cues				
Eat Mindfully & Slowly- Follow the 20 min meal				
Stop eating starchy carbs at 7pm				
Followed the 80/20 or 90/10 rule				
Any skipped meals				

Daily Exercise Plan

Activity	Length of W/O	Weight	Reps	Sets	Speed	Distance	Calories Burned

My Daily Reflections

Date:

Top 3 Daily Goals

My Action Steps To Help Me
Reach My Daily Goals Are:

- ______________________________
- ______________________________
- ______________________________

My Top 3 Strengths Are

Today I Found Happiness In

- ______________________________
- ______________________________
- ______________________________

3 Things I Love About My Body

I Am Grateful For

- ______________________________
- ______________________________
- ______________________________

Daily Meal Planner

MEAL PLAN		Macros Counts
Breakfast		Calories________ Carbs:________ Protein:______ Fats:________
Mid Morning		Calories________ Carbs:________ Protein:______ Fats:________
Lunch		Calories________ Carbs:________ Protein:______ Fats:________
Afternoon		Calories________ Carbs:________ Protein:______ Fats:________
Dinner		Calories________ Carbs:________ Protein:______ Fats:________

	Calories	Carbs	Protein	Fats
Calculated Macros				
Daily Totals				

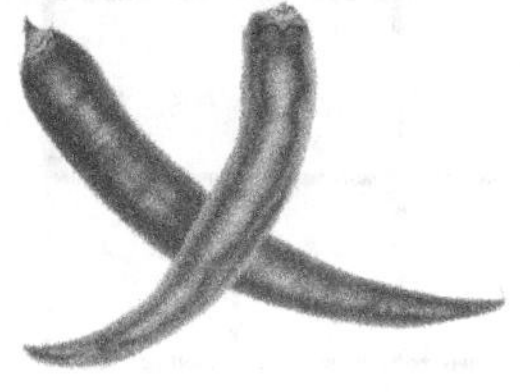
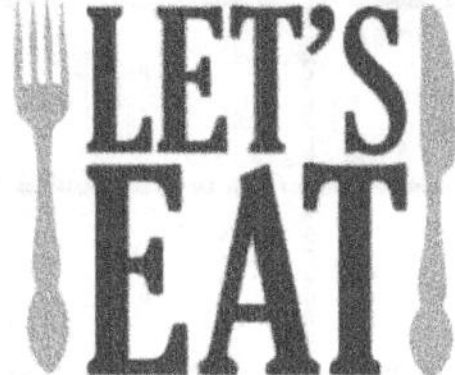

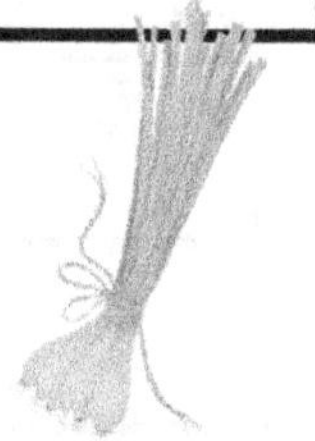

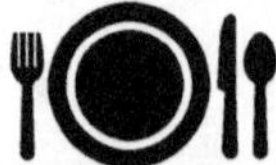 # Daily Healthy Eating Habits 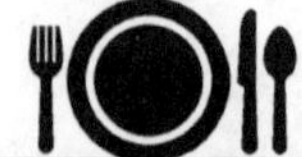

	Morning or Breakfast	Mid Day Or Lunch	Late Afternoon or Dinner	Evening Or Snacks
WATER- Drink 8-10 glasses or 3 L through out the day				
Veggies & Fruits- try to eat 5 servings each day				
Protein- Eat a palm size at each meal				
Healthy Fats- Eat fingertip - thumb size at each meal				
Follow Hand Portion Sizes at each meal				
Listen to Hunger & Fullness Cues				
Eat Mindfully & Slowly- Follow the 20 min meal				
Stop eating starchy carbs at 7pm				
Followed the 80/20 or 90/10 rule				
Any skipped meals				

Daily Exercise Plan

Activity	Length of W/O	Weight	Reps	Sets	Speed	Distance	Calories Burned

My Daily Reflections

Date:

⭐ Top 3 Daily Goals ⭐

☐ _______________________

☐ _______________________

☐ _______________________

My Action Steps To Help Me Reach My Daily Goals Are:

♥ My Top 3 Strengths Are ♥

☐ _______________________

☐ _______________________

☐ _______________________

Today I Found Happiness In

3 Things I Love About My Body

☐ _______________________

☐ _______________________

☐ _______________________

I Am Grateful For

Daily Meal Planner

MEAL PLAN		Macros Counts
Breakfast		Calories______ Carbs:______ Protein:______ Fats:______
Mid Morning		Calories______ Carbs:______ Protein:______ Fats:______
Lunch		Calories______ Carbs:______ Protein:______ Fats:______
Afternoon		Calories______ Carbs:______ Protein:______ Fats:______
Dinner		Calories______ Carbs:______ Protein:______ Fats:______

	Calories	Carbs	Protein	Fats
Calculated Macros				
Daily Totals				

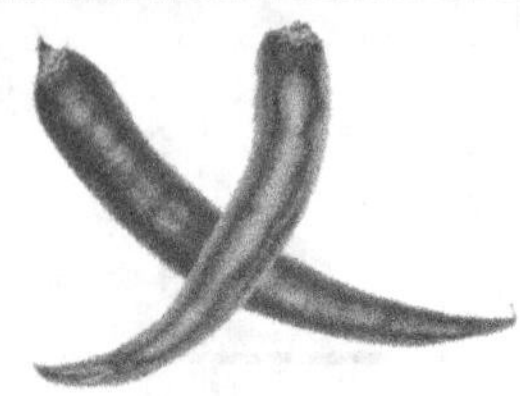
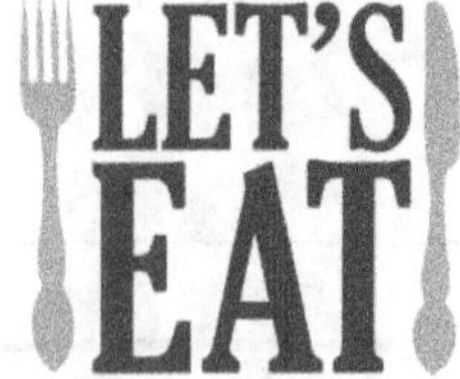

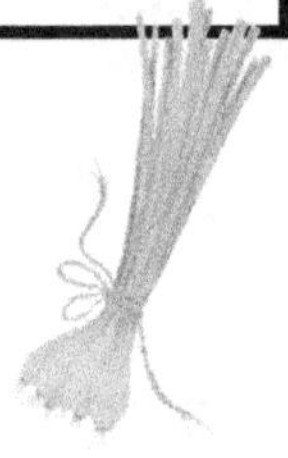

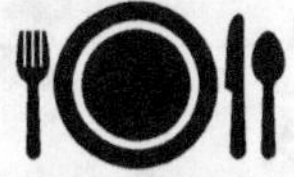 # Daily Healthy Eating Habits 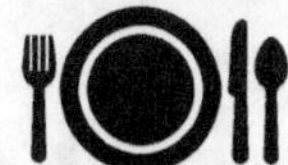

	Morning or Breakfast	Mid Day Or Lunch	Late Afternoon or Dinner	Evening Or Snacks
WATER- Drink 8-10 glasses or 3 L through out the day				
Veggies & Fruits- try to eat 5 servings each day				
Protein- Eat a palm size at each meal				
Healthy Fats- Eat fingertip - thumb size at each meal				
Follow Hand Portion Sizes at each meal				
Listen to Hunger & Fullness Cues				
Eat Mindfully & Slowly- Follow the 20 min meal				
Stop eating starchy carbs at 7pm				
Followed the 80/20 or 90/10 rule				
Any skipped meals				

Daily Exercise Plan

Activity	Length of W/O	Weight	Reps	Sets	Speed	Distance	Calories Burned

My Daily Reflections

Date:

★ Top 3 Daily Goals ★

My Action Steps To Help Me
Reach My Daily Goals Are:

- ☐ ___________________________
- ☐ ___________________________
- ☐ ___________________________

♥ My Top 3 Strengths Are ♥

Today I Found Happiness In

- ☐ ___________________________
- ☐ ___________________________
- ☐ ___________________________

3 Things I Love About My Body

I Am Grateful For

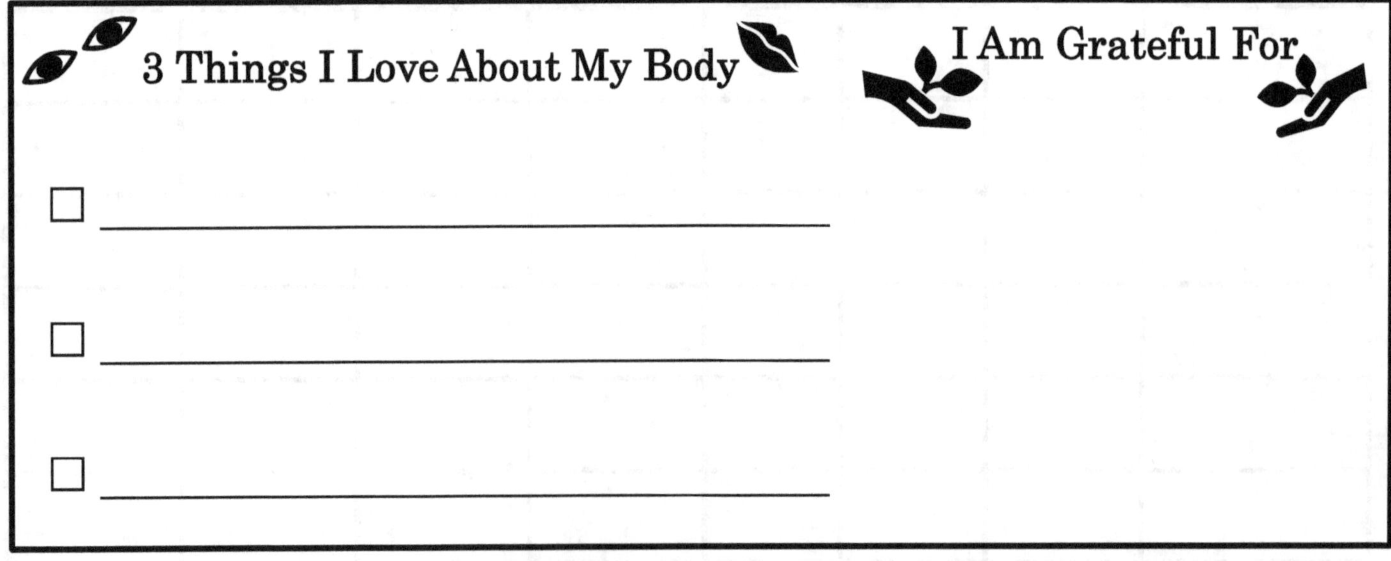

- ☐ ___________________________
- ☐ ___________________________
- ☐ ___________________________

Daily Meal Planner

MEAL PLAN		Macros Counts
Breakfast		Calories_______ Carbs:_______ Protein:_______ Fats:_________
Mid Morning		Calories_______ Carbs:_______ Protein:_______ Fats:_________
Lunch		Calories_______ Carbs:_______ Protein:_______ Fats:_________
Afternoon		Calories_______ Carbs:_______ Protein:_______ Fats:_________
Dinner		Calories_______ Carbs:_______ Protein:_______ Fats:_________

	Calories	Carbs	Protein	Fats
Calculated Macros				
Daily Totals				

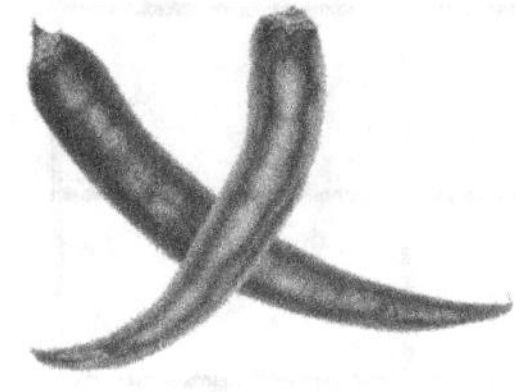
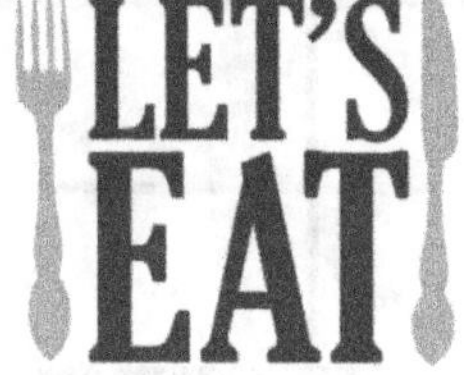

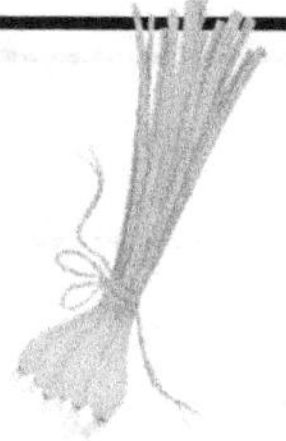

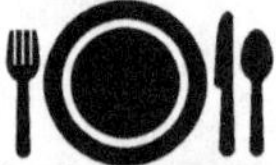 # Daily Healthy Eating Habits 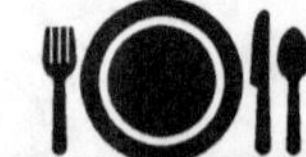

	Morning or Breakfast	Mid Day Or Lunch	Late Afternoon or Dinner	Evening Or Snacks
WATER- Drink 8-10 glasses or 3 L through out the day				
Veggies & Fruits- try to eat 5 servings each day				
Protein- Eat a palm size at each meal				
Healthy Fats- Eat fingertip - thumb size at each meal				
Follow Hand Portion Sizes at each meal				
Listen to Hunger & Fullness Cues				
Eat Mindfully & Slowly- Follow the 20 min meal				
Stop eating starchy carbs at 7pm				
Followed the 80/20 or 90/10 rule				
Any skipped meals				

Daily Exercise Plan

Activity	Length of W/O	Weight	Reps	Sets	Speed	Distance	Calories Burned

My Daily Reflections

Date:

★ Top 3 Daily Goals ★

My Action Steps To Help Me Reach My Daily Goals Are:

☐ ______________________________

☐ ______________________________

☐ ______________________________

♥ My Top 3 Strengths Are ♥

Today I Found Happiness In

☐ ______________________________

☐ ______________________________

☐ ______________________________

3 Things I Love About My Body

I Am Grateful For

☐ ______________________________

☐ ______________________________

☐ ______________________________

Daily Meal Planner

MEAL PLAN		Macros Counts
Breakfast		Calories________ Carbs:________ Protein:________ Fats:__________
Mid Morning		Calories________ Carbs:________ Protein:________ Fats:__________
Lunch		Calories________ Carbs:________ Protein:________ Fats:__________
Afternoon		Calories________ Carbs:________ Protein:________ Fats:__________
Dinner		Calories________ Carbs:________ Protein:________ Fats:__________

	Calories	Carbs	Protein	Fats
Calculated Macros				
Daily Totals				

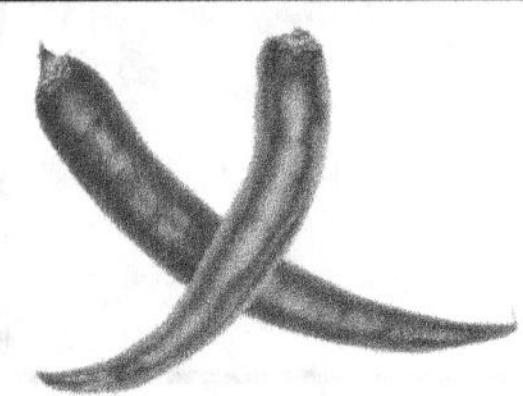

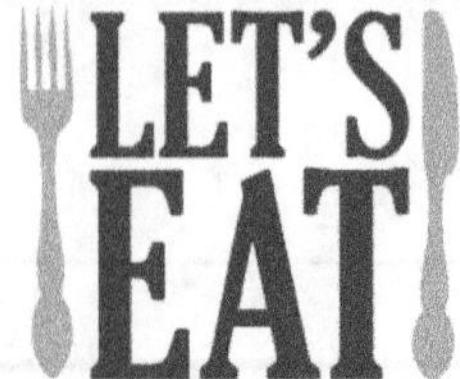

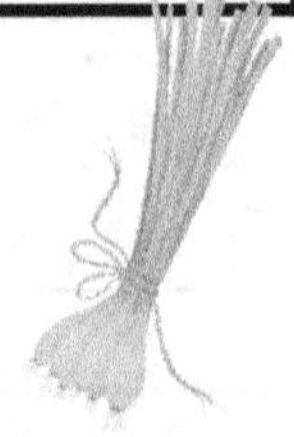

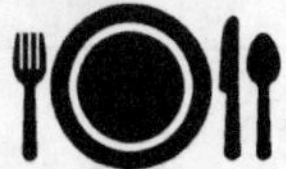 # Daily Healthy Eating Habits 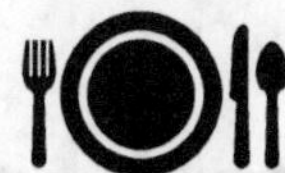

	Morning or Breakfast	Mid Day Or Lunch	Late Afternoon or Dinner	Evening Or Snacks
WATER- Drink 8-10 glasses or 3 L through out the day				
Veggies & Fruits- try to eat 5 servings each day				
Protein- Eat a palm size at each meal				
Healthy Fats- Eat fingertip - thumb size at each meal				
Follow Hand Portion Sizes at each meal				
Listen to Hunger & Fullness Cues				
Eat Mindfully & Slowly- Follow the 20 min meal				
Stop eating starchy carbs at 7pm				
Followed the 80/20 or 90/10 rule				
Any skipped meals				

Daily Exercise Plan

Activity	Length of W/O	Weight	Reps	Sets	Speed	Distance	Calories Burned

My Daily Reflections

Date:

Top 3 Daily Goals

My Action Steps To Help Me Reach My Daily Goals Are:

- [ ] ____________________
- [ ] ____________________
- [ ] ____________________

My Top 3 Strengths Are

Today I Found Happiness In

- [ ] ____________________
- [ ] ____________________
- [ ] ____________________

3 Things I Love About My Body

I Am Grateful For

- [ ] ____________________
- [ ] ____________________
- [ ] ____________________

Daily Meal Planner

MEAL PLAN	Macros Counts
Breakfast	Calories______ Carbs:______ Protein:______ Fats:______
Mid Morning	Calories______ Carbs:______ Protein:______ Fats:______
Lunch	Calories______ Carbs:______ Protein:______ Fats:______
Afternoon	Calories______ Carbs:______ Protein:______ Fats:______
Dinner	Calories______ Carbs:______ Protein:______ Fats:______

	Calories	Carbs	Protein	Fats
Calculated Macros				
Daily Totals				

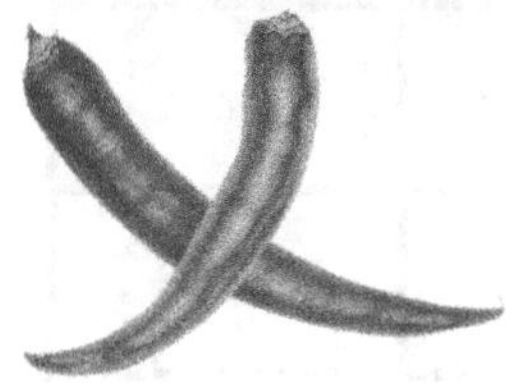
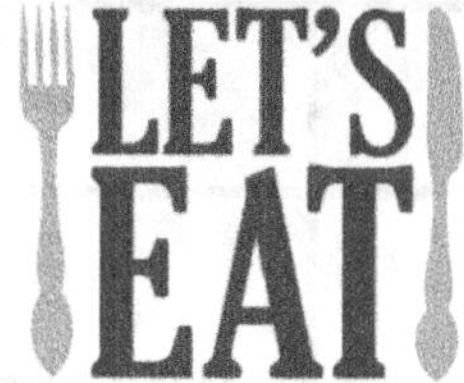

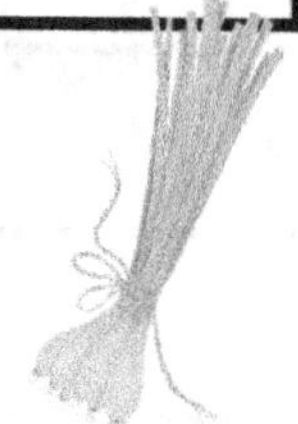

Daily Healthy Eating Habits

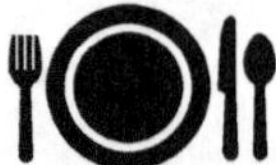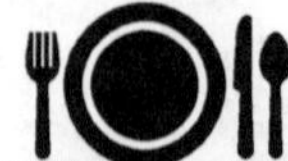

	Morning or Breakfast	Mid Day Or Lunch	Late Afternoon or Dinner	Evening Or Snacks
WATER- Drink 8-10 glasses or 3 L through out the day				
Veggies & Fruits- try to eat 5 servings each day				
Protein- Eat a palm size at each meal				
Healthy Fats- Eat fingertip - thumb size at each meal				
Follow Hand Portion Sizes at each meal				
Listen to Hunger & Fullness Cues				
Eat Mindfully & Slowly- Follow the 20 min meal				
Stop eating starchy carbs at 7pm				
Followed the 80/20 or 90/10 rule				
Any skipped meals				

Daily Exercise Plan

Activity	Length of W/O	Weight	Reps	Sets	Speed	Distance	Calories Burned

My Daily Reflections

Date:

Top 3 Daily Goals

- ☐ __________________________
- ☐ __________________________
- ☐ __________________________

My Action Steps To Help Me Reach My Daily Goals Are:

My Top 3 Strengths Are

- ☐ __________________________
- ☐ __________________________
- ☐ __________________________

Today I Found Happiness In

3 Things I Love About My Body

- ☐ __________________________
- ☐ __________________________
- ☐ __________________________

I Am Grateful For

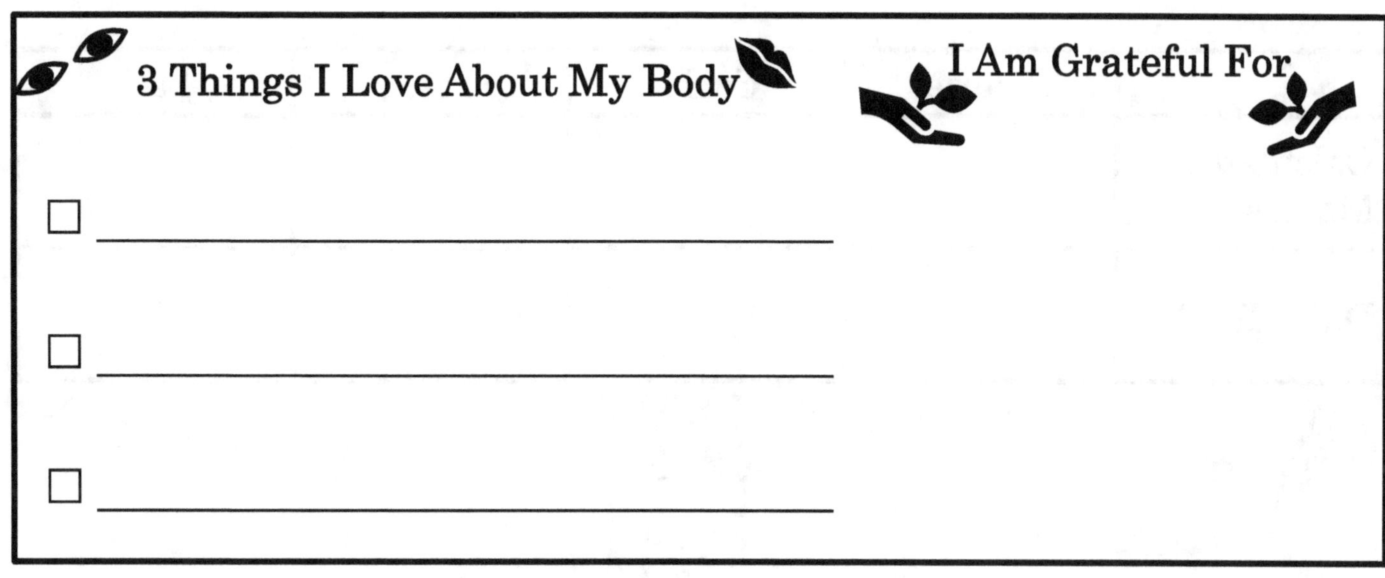

Daily Meal Planner

MEAL PLAN		Macros Counts
Breakfast		Calories________ Carbs:________ Protein:________ Fats:________
Mid Morning		Calories________ Carbs:________ Protein:________ Fats:________
Lunch		Calories________ Carbs:________ Protein:________ Fats:________
Afternoon		Calories________ Carbs:________ Protein:________ Fats:________
Dinner		Calories________ Carbs:________ Protein:________ Fats:________

	Calories	Carbs	Protein	Fats
Calculated Macros				
Daily Totals				

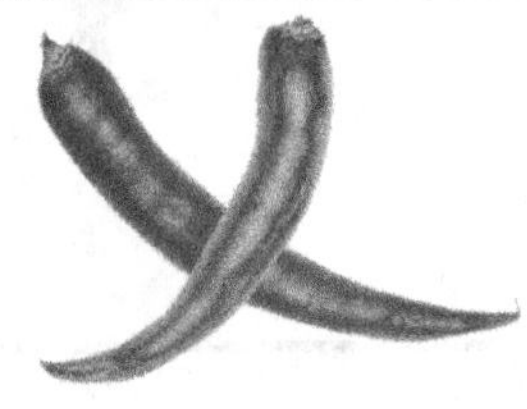

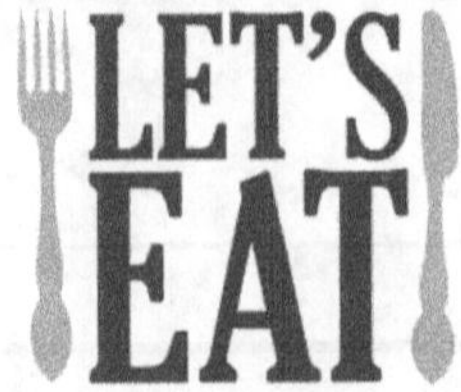

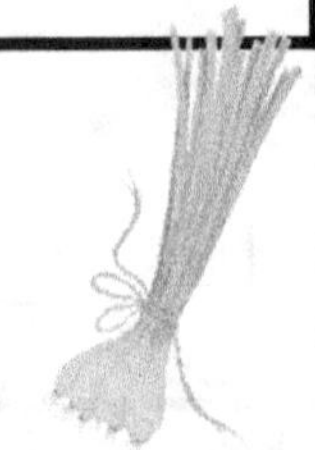

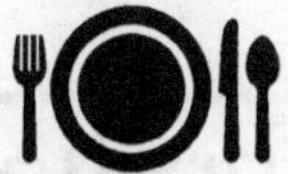 # Daily Healthy Eating Habits 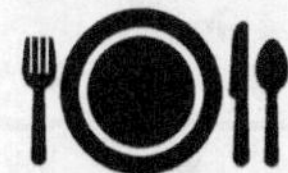

	Morning or Breakfast	Mid Day Or Lunch	Late Afternoon or Dinner	Evening Or Snacks
WATER- Drink 8-10 glasses or 3 L through out the day	⬦ ⬦ ⬦ ⬦ ⬦ ⬦ ⬦ ⬦			
Veggies & Fruits- try to eat 5 servings each day	🍎 🍎 🍎 🍎 🍎 🍎 🍎			
Protein- Eat a palm size at each meal				
Healthy Fats- Eat fingertip - thumb size at each meal				
Follow Hand Portion Sizes at each meal				
Listen to Hunger & Fullness Cues				
Eat Mindfully & Slowly- Follow the 20 min meal				
Stop eating starchy carbs at 7pm				
Followed the 80/20 or 90/10 rule				
Any skipped meals				

Daily Exercise Plan

Activity	Length of W/O	Weight	Reps	Sets	Speed	Distance	Calories Burned

<table>
<tr><td>Week Of:</td><td></td><td>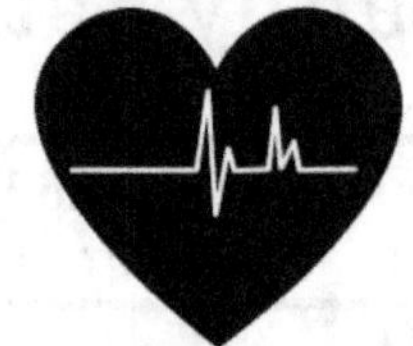</td><td colspan="2">Track Your Blood Sugar</td></tr>
</table>

Date	Wake Up	Pre-Lunch	Afternoon	Pre-Dinner	Bedtime

Results

High					
Good					
Low					

Note Any Changes

WEEK 11 FROM: _______________

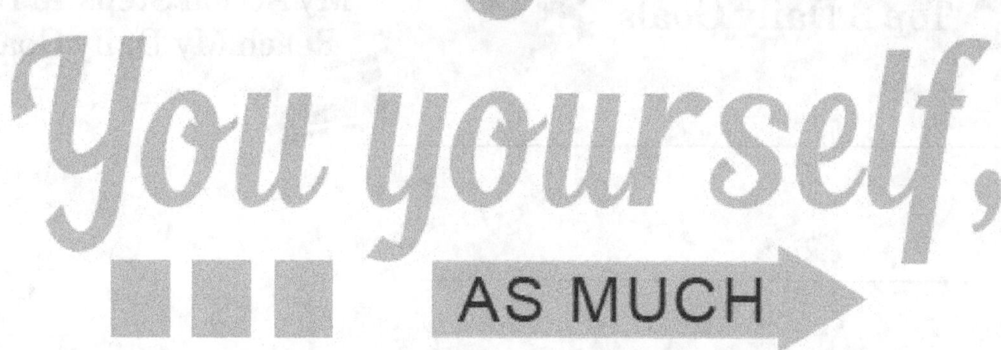

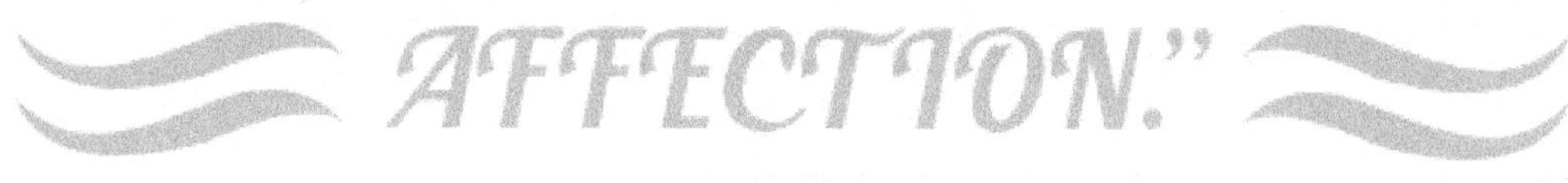

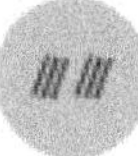

- Buddha

My Daily Reflections

Date:

⭐ Top 3 Daily Goals ⭐

My Action Steps To Help Me
Reach My Daily Goals Are:

- ☐ _______________________
- ☐ _______________________
- ☐ _______________________

♥ My Top 3 Strengths Are ♥

Today I Found Happiness In

- ☐ _______________________
- ☐ _______________________
- ☐ _______________________

3 Things I Love About My Body

I Am Grateful For

- ☐ _______________________
- ☐ _______________________
- ☐ _______________________

Daily Meal Planner

MEAL PLAN		Macros Counts
Breakfast		Calories_______ Carbs:_______ Protein:______ Fats:________
Mid Morning		Calories_______ Carbs:_______ Protein:______ Fats:________
Lunch		Calories_______ Carbs:_______ Protein:______ Fats:________
Afternoon		Calories_______ Carbs:_______ Protein:______ Fats:________
Dinner		Calories_______ Carbs:_______ Protein:______ Fats:________

	Calories	Carbs	Protein	Fats
Calculated Macros				
Daily Totals				

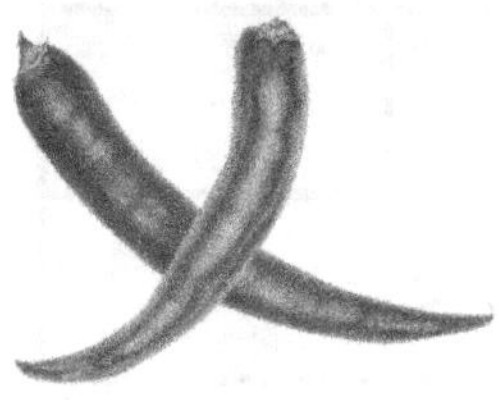

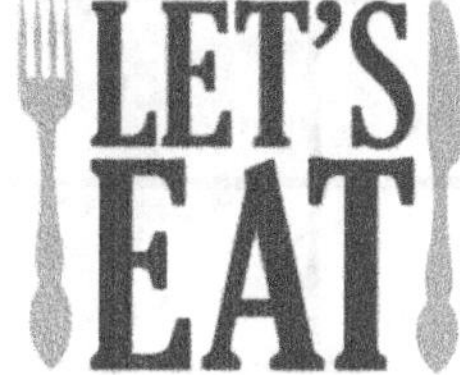

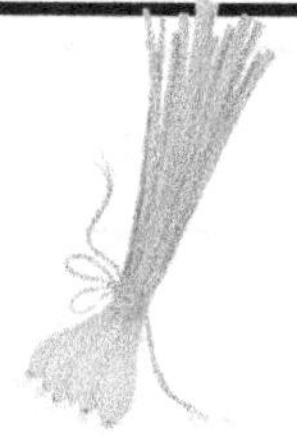

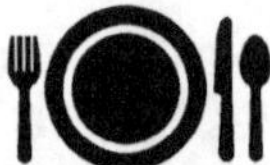 # Daily Healthy Eating Habits 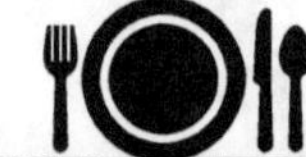

	Morning or Breakfast	Mid Day Or Lunch	Late Afternoon or Dinner	Evening Or Snacks
WATER- Drink 8-10 glasses or 3 L through out the day				
Veggies & Fruits- try to eat 5 servings each day				
Protein- Eat a palm size at each meal				
Healthy Fats- Eat fingertip - thumb size at each meal				
Follow Hand Portion Sizes at each meal				
Listen to Hunger & Fullness Cues				
Eat Mindfully & Slowly- Follow the 20 min meal				
Stop eating starchy carbs at 7pm				
Followed the 80/20 or 90/10 rule				
Any skipped meals				

Daily Exercise Plan

Activity	Length of W/O	Weight	Reps	Sets	Speed	Distance	Calories Burned

My Daily Reflections

Date:

★ Top 3 Daily Goals ★

☐ _______________

☐ _______________

☐ _______________

My Action Steps To Help Me Reach My Daily Goals Are:

♥ My Top 3 Strengths Are ♥

☐ _______________

☐ _______________

☐ _______________

Today I Found Happiness In

3 Things I Love About My Body

☐ _______________

☐ _______________

☐ _______________

I Am Grateful For

Daily Meal Planner

MEAL PLAN		Macros Counts
Breakfast		Calories______ Carbs:______ Protein:______ Fats:________
Mid Morning		Calories______ Carbs:______ Protein:______ Fats:________
Lunch		Calories______ Carbs:______ Protein:______ Fats:________
Afternoon		Calories______ Carbs:______ Protein:______ Fats:________
Dinner		Calories______ Carbs:______ Protein:______ Fats:________

	Calories	Carbs	Protein	Fats
Calculated Macros				
Daily Totals				

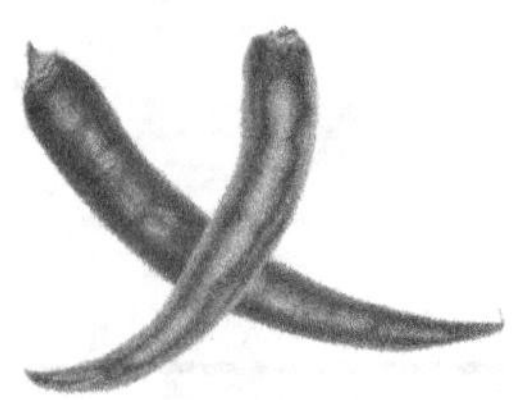
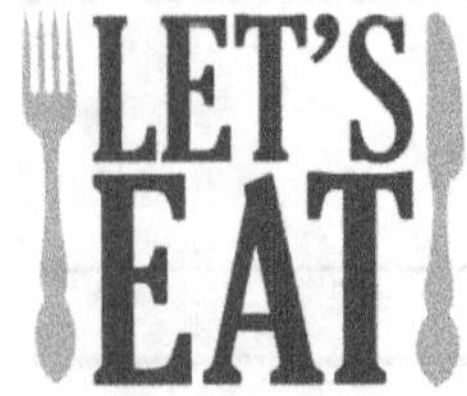

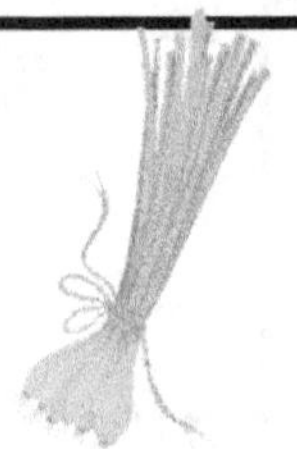

Daily Healthy Eating Habits

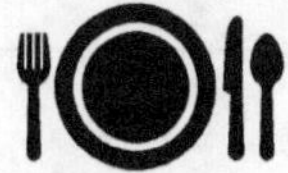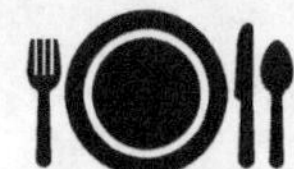

	Morning or Breakfast	Mid Day Or Lunch	Late Afternoon or Dinner	Evening Or Snacks
WATER- Drink 8-10 glasses or 3 L through out the day				
Veggies & Fruits- try to eat 5 servings each day				
Protein- Eat a palm size at each meal				
Healthy Fats- Eat fingertip - thumb size at each meal				
Follow Hand Portion Sizes at each meal				
Listen to Hunger & Fullness Cues				
Eat Mindfully & Slowly- Follow the 20 min meal				
Stop eating starchy carbs at 7pm				
Followed the 80/20 or 90/10 rule				
Any skipped meals				

Daily Exercise Plan

Activity	Length of W/O	Weight	Reps	Sets	Speed	Distance	Calories Burned

My Daily Reflections

Date:

⭐ Top 3 Daily Goals ⭐

- ☐ _______________________________
- ☐ _______________________________
- ☐ _______________________________

My Action Steps To Help Me Reach My Daily Goals Are:

♥ My Top 3 Strengths Are ♥

- ☐ _______________________________
- ☐ _______________________________
- ☐ _______________________________

Today I Found Happiness In

3 Things I Love About My Body

- ☐ _______________________________
- ☐ _______________________________
- ☐ _______________________________

I Am Grateful For

Daily Meal Planner

MEAL PLAN		Macros Counts
Breakfast		Calories______ Carbs:______ Protein:______ Fats:________
Mid Morning		Calories______ Carbs:______ Protein:______ Fats:________
Lunch		Calories______ Carbs:______ Protein:______ Fats:________
Afternoon		Calories______ Carbs:______ Protein:______ Fats:________
Dinner		Calories______ Carbs:______ Protein:______ Fats:________

	Calories	Carbs	Protein	Fats
Calculated Macros				
Daily Totals				

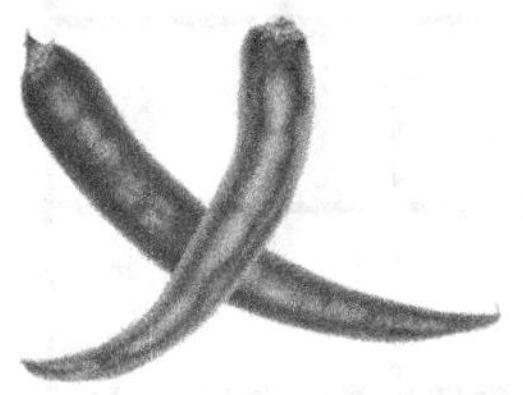

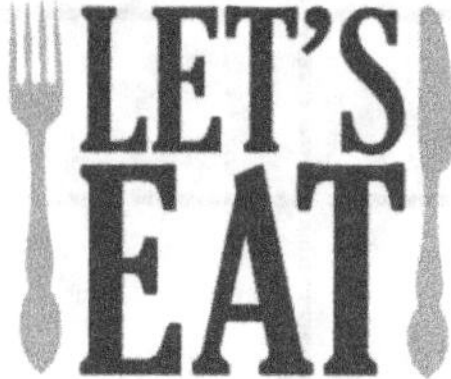

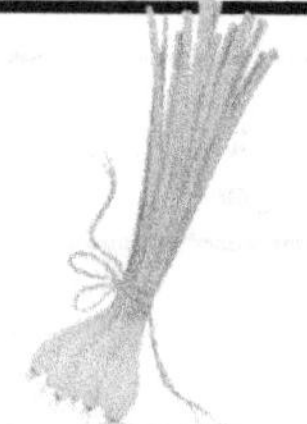

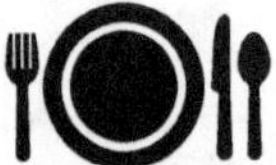 # Daily Healthy Eating Habits 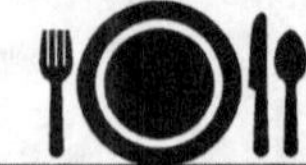

	Morning or Breakfast	Mid Day Or Lunch	Late Afternoon or Dinner	Evening Or Snacks
WATER- Drink 8-10 glasses or 3 L through out the day				
Veggies & Fruits- try to eat 5 servings each day				
Protein- Eat a palm size at each meal				
Healthy Fats- Eat fingertip - thumb size at each meal				
Follow Hand Portion Sizes at each meal				
Listen to Hunger & Fullness Cues				
Eat Mindfully & Slowly- Follow the 20 min meal				
Stop eating starchy carbs at 7pm				
Followed the 80/20 or 90/10 rule				
Any skipped meals				

Daily Exercise Plan

Activity	Length of W/O	Weight	Reps	Sets	Speed	Distance	Calories Burned

My Daily Reflections

Date:

★ Top 3 Daily Goals ★

☐ _______________________

☐ _______________________

☐ _______________________

My Action Steps To Help Me Reach My Daily Goals Are:

♥ My Top 3 Strengths Are ♥

☐ _______________________

☐ _______________________

☐ _______________________

Today I Found Happiness In

3 Things I Love About My Body

☐ _______________________

☐ _______________________

☐ _______________________

I Am Grateful For

Daily Meal Planner

MEAL PLAN		Macros Counts
Breakfast		Calories________ Carbs:________ Protein:______ Fats:__________
Mid Morning		Calories________ Carbs:________ Protein:______ Fats:__________
Lunch		Calories________ Carbs:________ Protein:______ Fats:__________
Afternoon		Calories________ Carbs:________ Protein:______ Fats:__________
Dinner		Calories________ Carbs:________ Protein:______ Fats:__________

	Calories	Carbs	Protein	Fats
Calculated Macros				
Daily Totals				

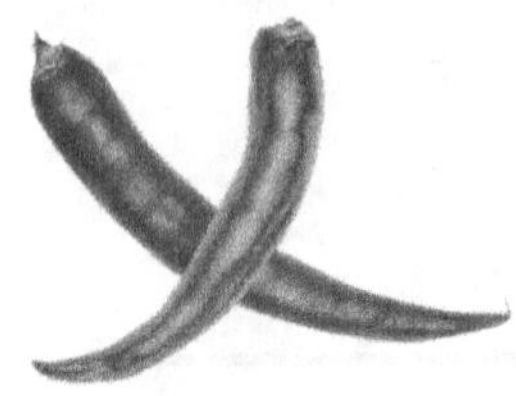

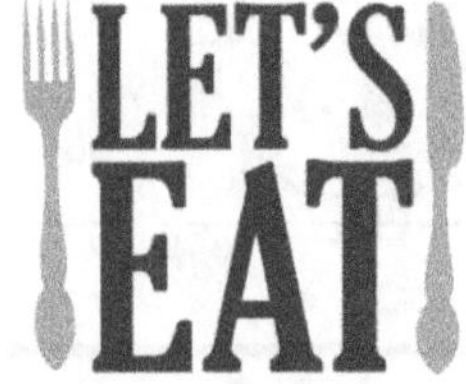

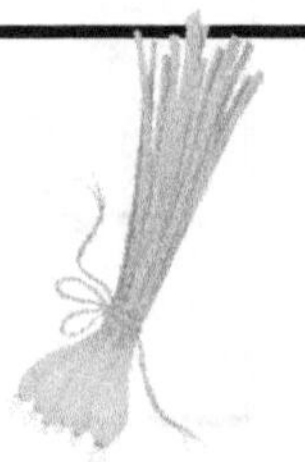

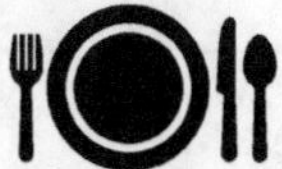 # Daily Healthy Eating Habits 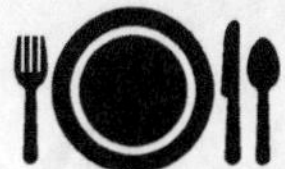

	Morning or Breakfast	Mid Day Or Lunch	Late Afternoon or Dinner	Evening Or Snacks
WATER- Drink 8-10 glasses or 3 L through out the day				
Veggies & Fruits- try to eat 5 servings each day				
Protein- Eat a palm size at each meal				
Healthy Fats- Eat fingertip - thumb size at each meal				
Follow Hand Portion Sizes at each meal				
Listen to Hunger & Fullness Cues				
Eat Mindfully & Slowly- Follow the 20 min meal				
Stop eating starchy carbs at 7pm				
Followed the 80/20 or 90/10 rule				
Any skipped meals				

Daily Exercise Plan

Activity	Length of W/O	Weight	Reps	Sets	Speed	Distance	Calories Burned

My Daily Reflections

Top 3 Daily Goals

- ☐ ___________________________
- ☐ ___________________________
- ☐ ___________________________

My Action Steps To Help Me Reach My Daily Goals Are:

My Top 3 Strengths Are

- ☐ ___________________________
- ☐ ___________________________
- ☐ ___________________________

Today I Found Happiness In

3 Things I Love About My Body

- ☐ ___________________________
- ☐ ___________________________
- ☐ ___________________________

I Am Grateful For

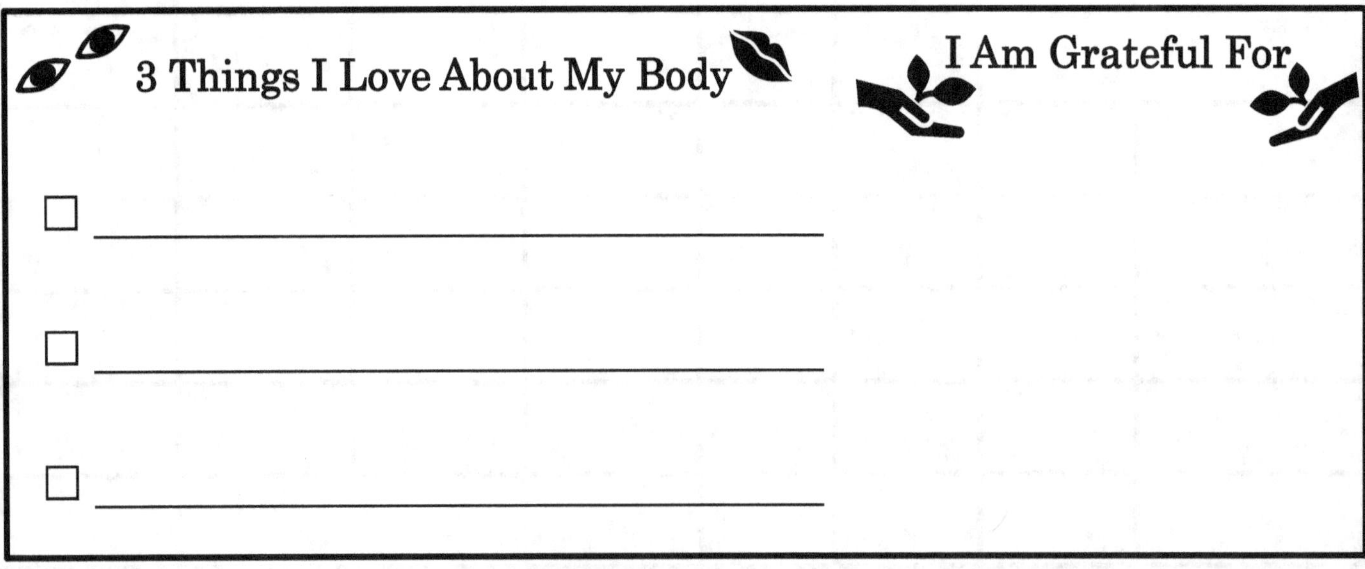

Daily Meal Planner

MEAL PLAN		Macros Counts
Breakfast		Calories________ Carbs:________ Protein:________ Fats:________
Mid Morning		Calories________ Carbs:________ Protein:________ Fats:________
Lunch		Calories________ Carbs:________ Protein:________ Fats:________
Afternoon		Calories________ Carbs:________ Protein:________ Fats:________
Dinner		Calories________ Carbs:________ Protein:________ Fats:________

	Calories	Carbs	Protein	Fats
Calculated Macros				
Daily Totals				

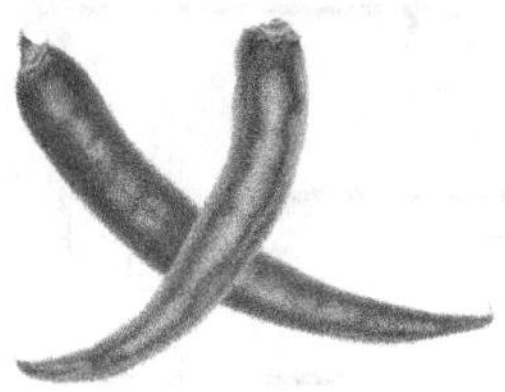
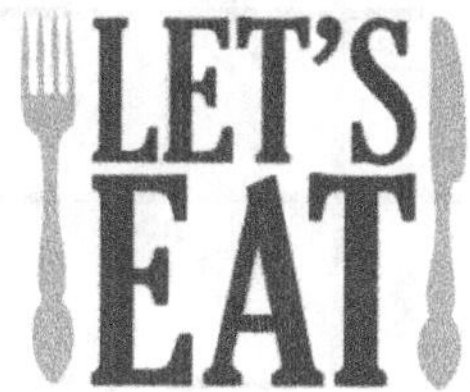

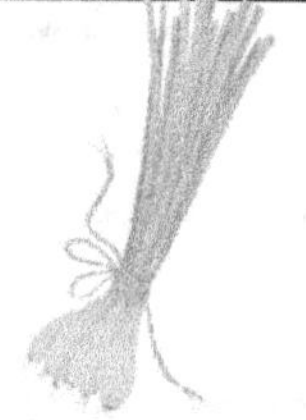

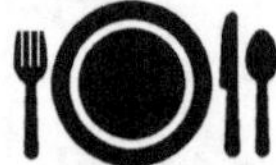 # Daily Healthy Eating Habits 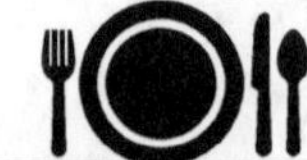

	Morning or Breakfast	Mid Day Or Lunch	Late Afternoon or Dinner	Evening Or Snacks
WATER- Drink 8-10 glasses or 3 L through out the day				
Veggies & Fruits- try to eat 5 servings each day				
Protein- Eat a palm size at each meal				
Healthy Fats- Eat fingertip - thumb size at each meal				
Follow Hand Portion Sizes at each meal				
Listen to Hunger & Fullness Cues				
Eat Mindfully & Slowly- Follow the 20 min meal				
Stop eating starchy carbs at 7pm				
Followed the 80/20 or 90/10 rule				
Any skipped meals				

Daily Exercise Plan

Activity	Length of W/O	Weight	Reps	Sets	Speed	Distance	Calories Burned

My Daily Reflections

Date:

⭐ Top 3 Daily Goals ⭐

My Action Steps To Help Me
Reach My Daily Goals Are:

- [ ] ___________________________
- [ ] ___________________________
- [ ] ___________________________

♥ My Top 3 Strengths Are ♥

Today I Found Happiness In

- [ ] ___________________________
- [ ] ___________________________
- [ ] ___________________________

3 Things I Love About My Body

I Am Grateful For

- [ ] ___________________________
- [ ] ___________________________
- [ ] ___________________________

Daily Meal Planner

MEAL PLAN	Macros Counts
Breakfast	Calories_______ Carbs:_______ Protein:_______ Fats:_________
Mid Morning	Calories_______ Carbs:_______ Protein:_______ Fats:_________
Lunch	Calories_______ Carbs:_______ Protein:_______ Fats:_________
Afternoon	Calories_______ Carbs:_______ Protein:_______ Fats:_________
Dinner	Calories_______ Carbs:_______ Protein:_______ Fats:_________

	Calories	Carbs	Protein	Fats
Calculated Macros				
Daily Totals				

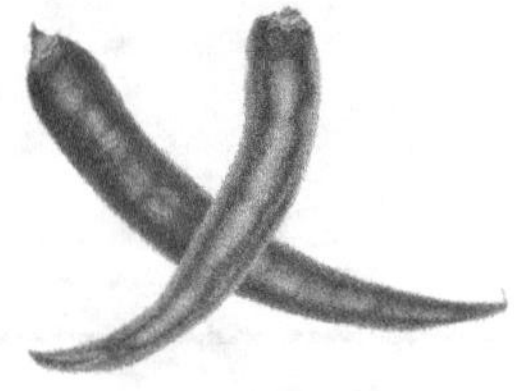
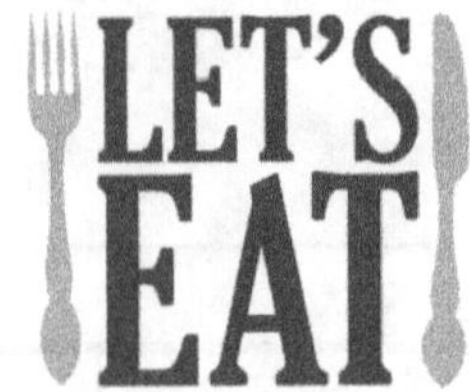

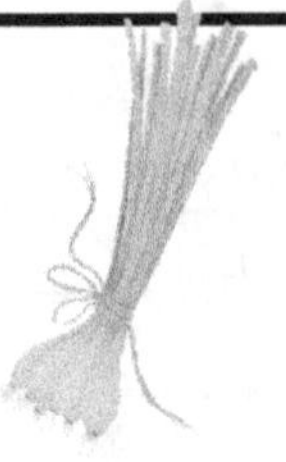

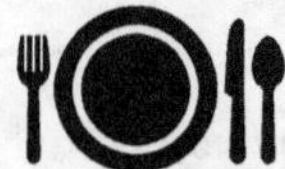 # Daily Healthy Eating Habits 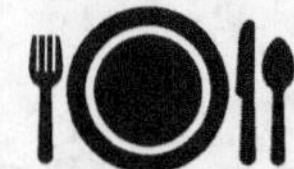

	Morning or Breakfast	Mid Day Or Lunch	Late Afternoon or Dinner	Evening Or Snacks
WATER- Drink 8-10 glasses or 3 L through out the day				
Veggies & Fruits- try to eat 5 servings each day				
Protein- Eat a palm size at each meal				
Healthy Fats- Eat fingertip - thumb size at each meal				
Follow Hand Portion Sizes at each meal				
Listen to Hunger & Fullness Cues				
Eat Mindfully & Slowly- Follow the 20 min meal				
Stop eating starchy carbs at 7pm				
Followed the 80/20 or 90/10 rule				
Any skipped meals				

Daily Exercise Plan

Activity	Length of W/O	Weight	Reps	Sets	Speed	Distance	Calories Burned

My Daily Reflections

Date:

⭐ Top 3 Daily Goals ⭐

☐ __________________________

☐ __________________________

☐ __________________________

My Action Steps To Help Me Reach My Daily Goals Are:

♥ My Top 3 Strengths Are ♥

☐ __________________________

☐ __________________________

☐ __________________________

Today I Found Happiness In

3 Things I Love About My Body

☐ __________________________

☐ __________________________

☐ __________________________

I Am Grateful For

Daily Meal Planner

MEAL PLAN		Macros Counts
Breakfast		Calories______ Carbs:______ Protein:______ Fats:______
Mid Morning		Calories______ Carbs:______ Protein:______ Fats:______
Lunch		Calories______ Carbs:______ Protein:______ Fats:______
Afternoon		Calories______ Carbs:______ Protein:______ Fats:______
Dinner		Calories______ Carbs:______ Protein:______ Fats:______

	Calories	Carbs	Protein	Fats
Calculated Macros				
Daily Totals				

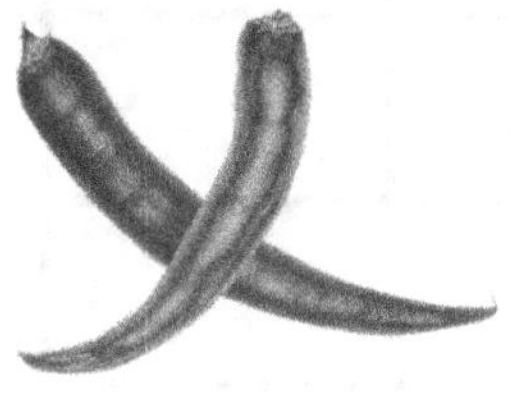

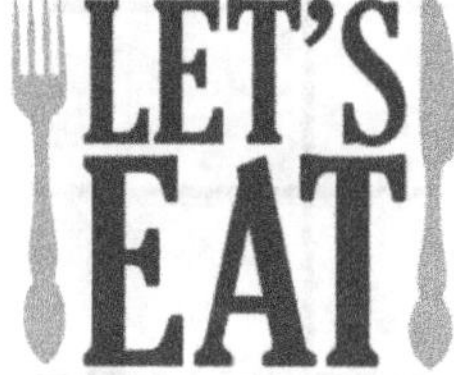

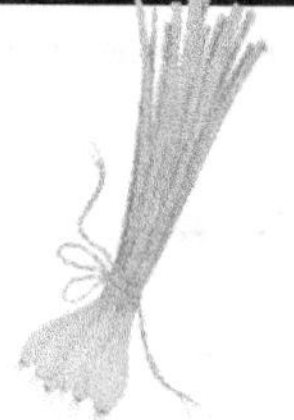

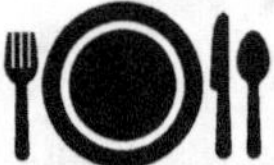 # Daily Healthy Eating Habits 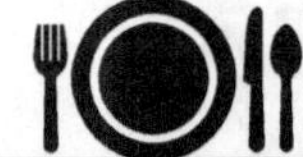

	Morning or Breakfast	Mid Day Or Lunch	Late Afternoon or Dinner	Evening Or Snacks
WATER- Drink 8-10 glasses or 3 L through out the day				
Veggies & Fruits- try to eat 5 servings each day				
Protein- Eat a palm size at each meal				
Healthy Fats- Eat fingertip - thumb size at each meal				
Follow Hand Portion Sizes at each meal				
Listen to Hunger & Fullness Cues				
Eat Mindfully & Slowly- Follow the 20 min meal				
Stop eating starchy carbs at 7pm				
Followed the 80/20 or 90/10 rule				
Any skipped meals				

Daily Exercise Plan

Activity	Length of W/O	Weight	Reps	Sets	Speed	Distance	Calories Burned

<table>
<tr><td>

Week Of:

</td><td>

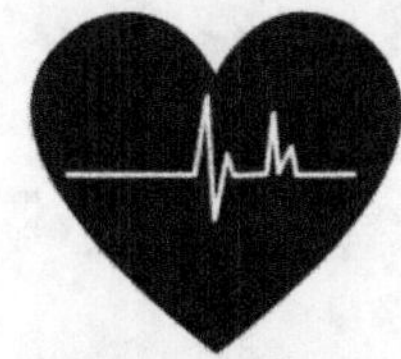

</td><td>

Track Your Blood Sugar

</td></tr>
</table>

Date	Wake Up	Pre-Lunch	Afternoon	Pre-Dinner	Bedtime

Results

High				
Good				
Low				

Note Any Changes

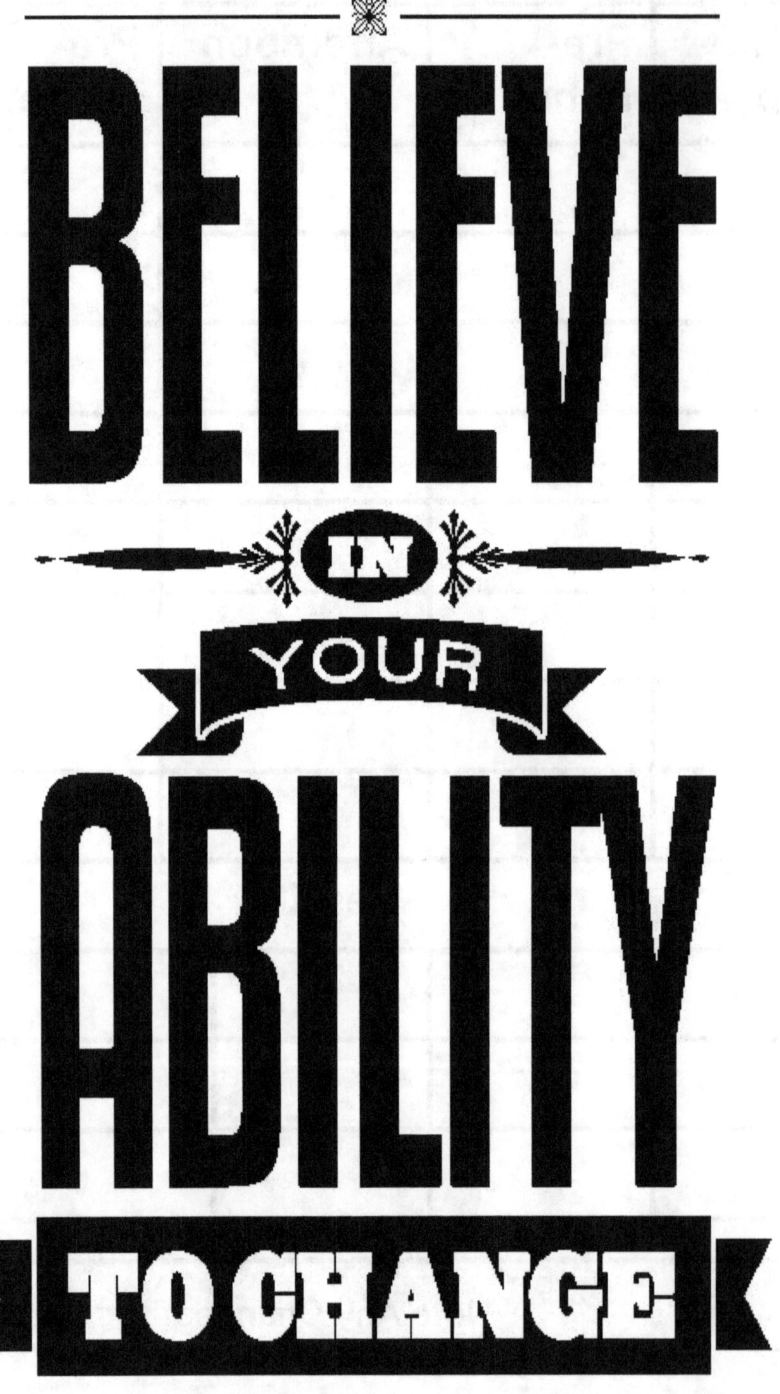

BREAKING BAD HABITS

My Daily Reflections

Date:

⭐ Top 3 Daily Goals ⭐

- ☐ __________________________
- ☐ __________________________
- ☐ __________________________

My Action Steps To Help Me Reach My Daily Goals Are:

♥ My Top 3 Strengths Are ♥

- ☐ __________________________
- ☐ __________________________
- ☐ __________________________

Today I Found Happiness In

3 Things I Love About My Body

- ☐ __________________________
- ☐ __________________________
- ☐ __________________________

I Am Grateful For

Daily Meal Planner

MEAL PLAN		Macros Counts
Breakfast		Calories_______ Carbs:_______ Protein:______ Fats:_________
Mid Morning		Calories_______ Carbs:_______ Protein:______ Fats:_________
Lunch		Calories_______ Carbs:_______ Protein:______ Fats:_________
Afternoon		Calories_______ Carbs:_______ Protein:______ Fats:_________
Dinner		Calories_______ Carbs:_______ Protein:______ Fats:_________

	Calories	Carbs	Protein	Fats
Calculated Macros				
Daily Totals				

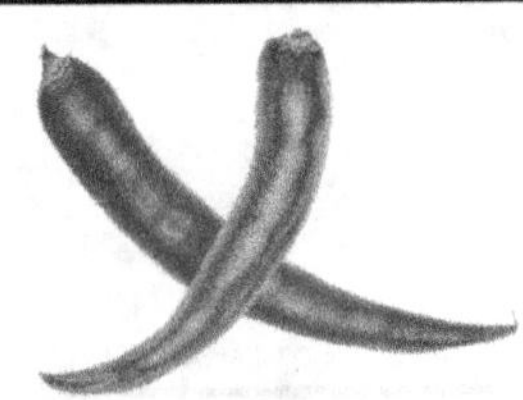
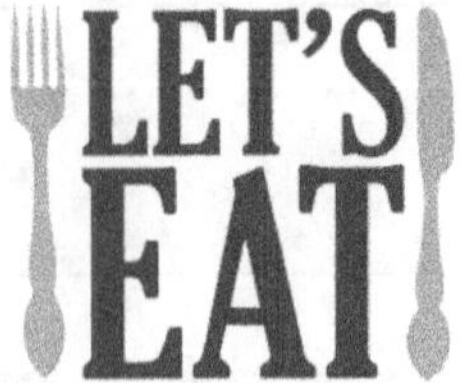

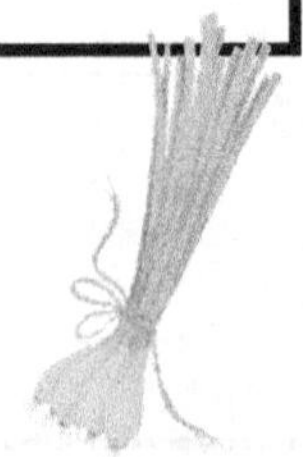

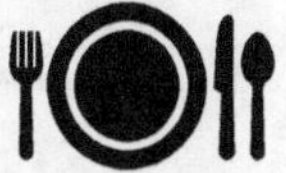 # Daily Healthy Eating Habits 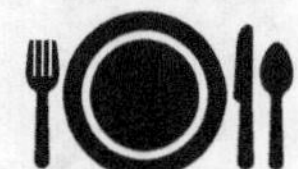

	Morning or Breakfast	Mid Day Or Lunch	Late Afternoon or Dinner	Evening Or Snacks
WATER- Drink 8-10 glasses or 3 L through out the day				
Veggies & Fruits- try to eat 5 servings each day				
Protein- Eat a palm size at each meal				
Healthy Fats- Eat fingertip - thumb size at each meal				
Follow Hand Portion Sizes at each meal				
Listen to Hunger & Fullness Cues				
Eat Mindfully & Slowly- Follow the 20 min meal				
Stop eating starchy carbs at 7pm				
Followed the 80/20 or 90/10 rule				
Any skipped meals				

Daily Exercise Plan

Activity	Length of W/O	Weight	Reps	Sets	Speed	Distance	Calories Burned

My Daily Reflections

Date:

Top 3 Daily Goals

My Action Steps To Help Me Reach My Daily Goals Are:

- [ ]
- [ ]
- [ ]

My Top 3 Strengths Are

Today I Found Happiness In

- [ ]
- [ ]
- [ ]

3 Things I Love About My Body

I Am Grateful For

- [ ]
- [ ]
- [ ]

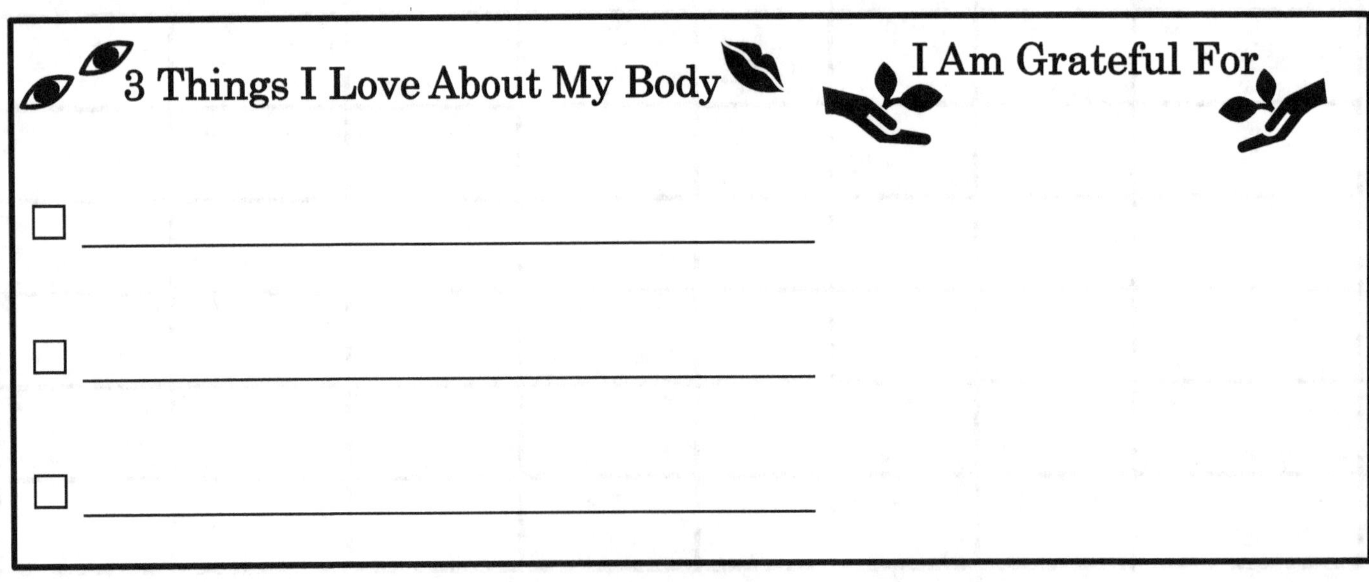

Daily Meal Planner

MEAL PLAN		Macros Counts
Breakfast		Calories________ Carbs:_________ Protein:_______ Fats:__________
Mid Morning		Calories________ Carbs:_________ Protein:_______ Fats:__________
Lunch		Calories________ Carbs:_________ Protein:_______ Fats:__________
Afternoon		Calories________ Carbs:_________ Protein:_______ Fats:__________
Dinner		Calories________ Carbs:_________ Protein:_______ Fats:__________

	Calories	Carbs	Protein	Fats
Calculated Macros				
Daily Totals				

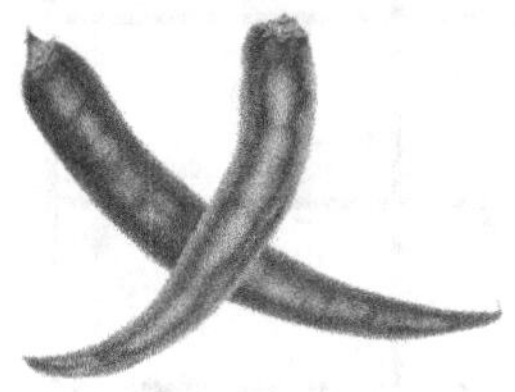

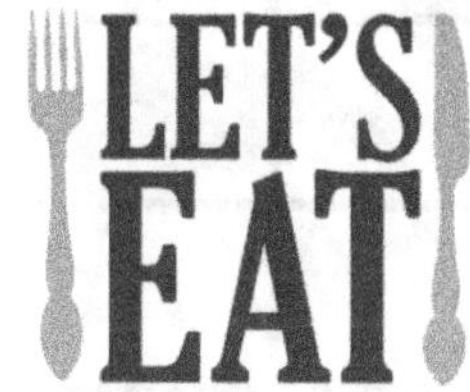

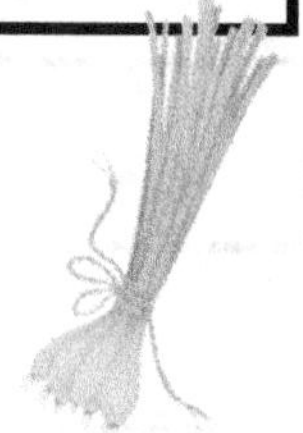

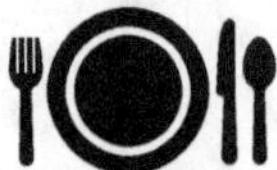 # Daily Healthy Eating Habits 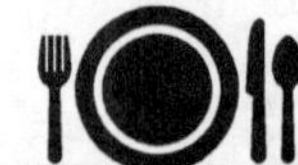

	Morning or Breakfast	Mid Day Or Lunch	Late Afternoon or Dinner	Evening Or Snacks
WATER- Drink 8-10 glasses or 3 L through out the day				
Veggies & Fruits- try to eat 5 servings each day				
Protein- Eat a palm size at each meal				
Healthy Fats- Eat fingertip - thumb size at each meal				
Follow Hand Portion Sizes at each meal				
Listen to Hunger & Fullness Cues				
Eat Mindfully & Slowly- Follow the 20 min meal				
Stop eating starchy carbs at 7pm				
Followed the 80/20 or 90/10 rule				
Any skipped meals				

Daily Exercise Plan

Activity	Length of W/O	Weight	Reps	Sets	Speed	Distance	Calories Burned

My Daily Reflections

Date:

Top 3 Daily Goals

☐ ___________________________

☐ ___________________________

☐ ___________________________

My Action Steps To Help Me Reach My Daily Goals Are:

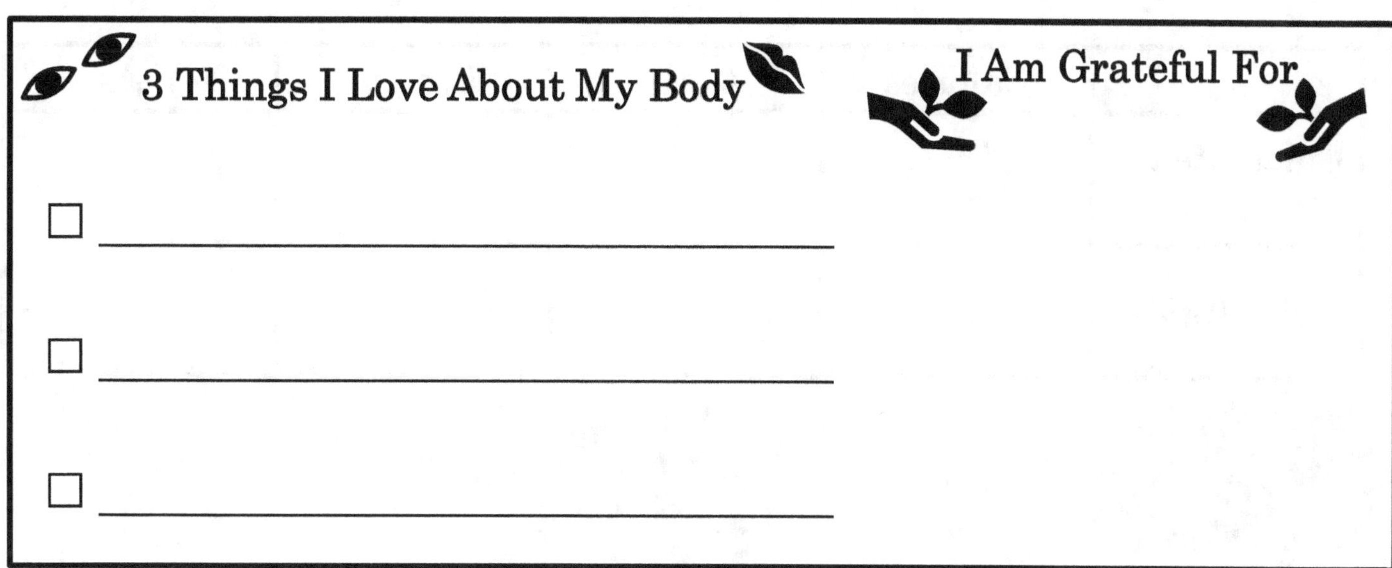

My Top 3 Strengths Are

☐ ___________________________

☐ ___________________________

☐ ___________________________

Today I Found Happiness In

3 Things I Love About My Body

☐ ___________________________

☐ ___________________________

☐ ___________________________

I Am Grateful For

Daily Meal Planner

MEAL PLAN		Macros Counts
Breakfast		Calories________ Carbs:________ Protein:______ Fats:__________
Mid Morning		Calories________ Carbs:________ Protein:______ Fats:__________
Lunch		Calories________ Carbs:________ Protein:______ Fats:__________
Afternoon		Calories________ Carbs:________ Protein:______ Fats:__________
Dinner		Calories________ Carbs:________ Protein:______ Fats:__________

	Calories	Carbs	Protein	Fats
Calculated Macros				
Daily Totals				

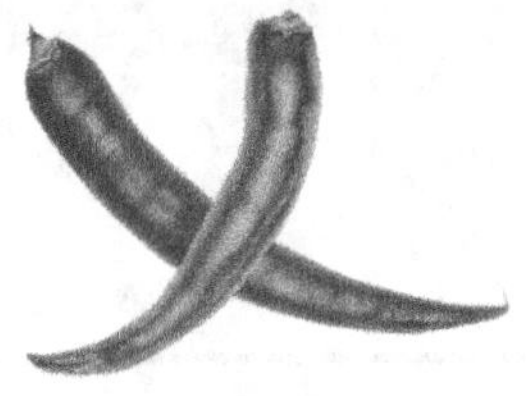

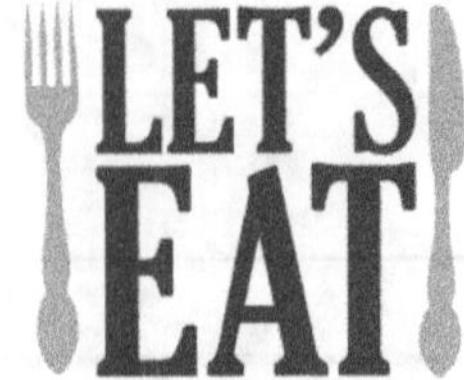

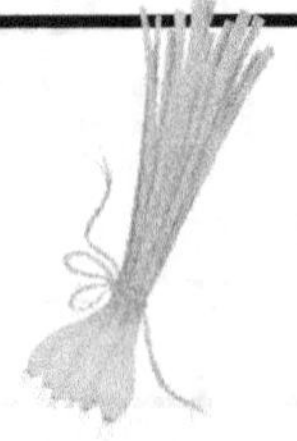

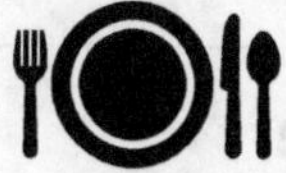 # Daily Healthy Eating Habits 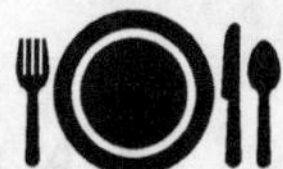

	Morning or Breakfast	Mid Day Or Lunch	Late Afternoon or Dinner	Evening Or Snacks
WATER- Drink 8-10 glasses or 3 L through out the day				
Veggies & Fruits- try to eat 5 servings each day				
Protein- Eat a palm size at each meal				
Healthy Fats- Eat fingertip - thumb size at each meal				
Follow Hand Portion Sizes at each meal				
Listen to Hunger & Fullness Cues				
Eat Mindfully & Slowly- Follow the 20 min meal				
Stop eating starchy carbs at 7pm				
Followed the 80/20 or 90/10 rule				
Any skipped meals				

Daily Exercise Plan

Activity	Length of W/O	Weight	Reps	Sets	Speed	Distance	Calories Burned

My Daily Reflections

Date:

Top 3 Daily Goals

- ☐ _______________________
- ☐ _______________________
- ☐ _______________________

My Action Steps To Help Me Reach My Daily Goals Are:

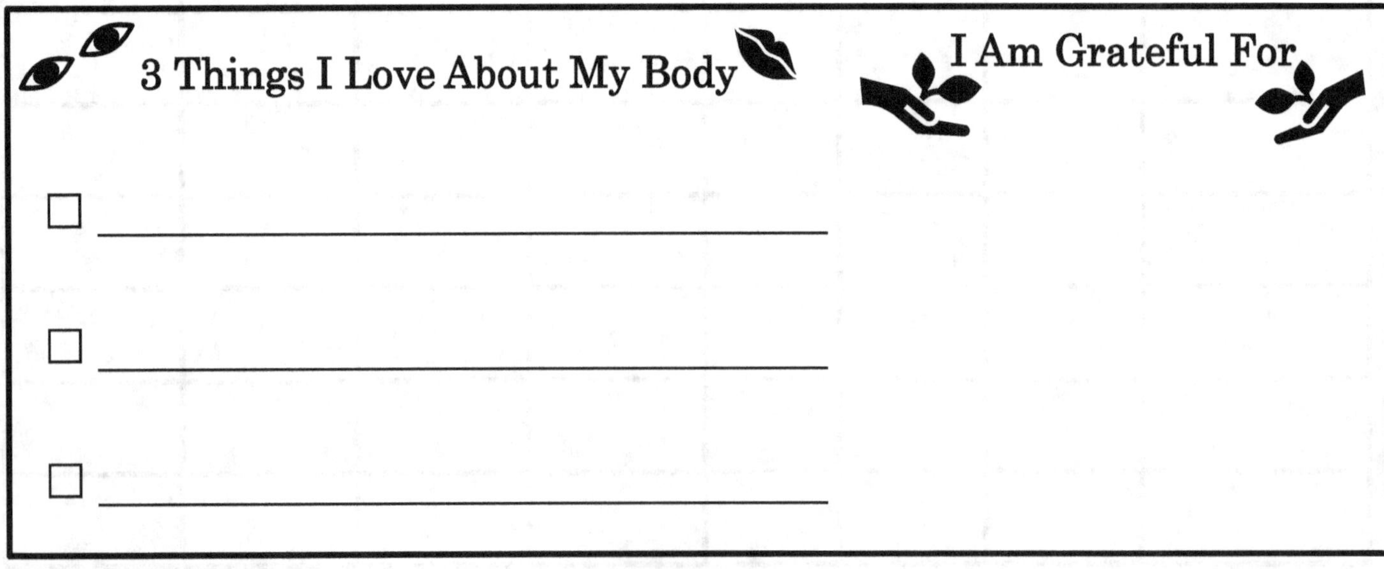

My Top 3 Strengths Are

- ☐ _______________________
- ☐ _______________________
- ☐ _______________________

Today I Found Happiness In

3 Things I Love About My Body

- ☐ _______________________
- ☐ _______________________
- ☐ _______________________

I Am Grateful For

Daily Meal Planner

MEAL PLAN		Macros Counts
Breakfast		Calories________ Carbs:________ Protein:______ Fats:________
Mid Morning		Calories________ Carbs:______ Protein:______ Fats:________
Lunch		Calories______ Carbs:______ Protein:______ Fats:________
Afternoon		Calories______ Carbs:________ Protein:______ Fats:________
Dinner		Calories______ Carbs:______ Protein:______ Fats:________

	Calories	Carbs	Protein	Fats
Calculated Macros				
Daily Totals				

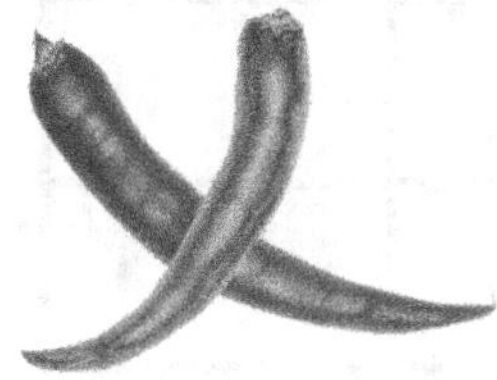

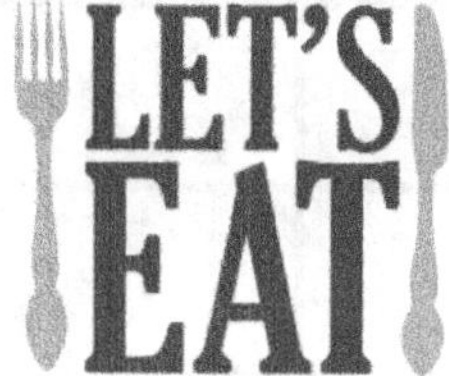

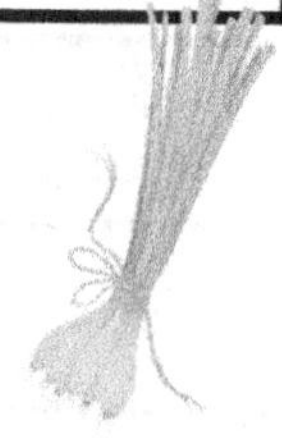

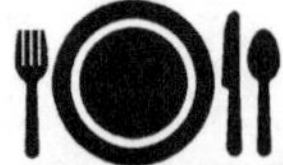 # Daily Healthy Eating Habits 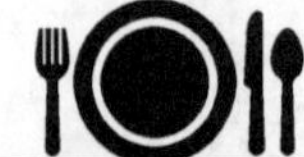

	Morning or Breakfast	Mid Day Or Lunch	Late Afternoon or Dinner	Evening Or Snacks
WATER- Drink 8-10 glasses or 3 L through out the day				
Veggies & Fruits- try to eat 5 servings each day				
Protein- Eat a palm size at each meal				
Healthy Fats- Eat fingertip - thumb size at each meal				
Follow Hand Portion Sizes at each meal				
Listen to Hunger & Fullness Cues				
Eat Mindfully & Slowly- Follow the 20 min meal				
Stop eating starchy carbs at 7pm				
Followed the 80/20 or 90/10 rule				
Any skipped meals				

Daily Exercise Plan

Activity	Length of W/O	Weight	Reps	Sets	Speed	Distance	Calories Burned

My Daily Reflections

Date:

★ Top 3 Daily Goals ★

- ☐ __________________________
- ☐ __________________________
- ☐ __________________________

My Action Steps To Help Me Reach My Daily Goals Are:

♥ My Top 3 Strengths Are ♥

- ☐ __________________________
- ☐ __________________________
- ☐ __________________________

Today I Found Happiness In

3 Things I Love About My Body

- ☐ __________________________
- ☐ __________________________
- ☐ __________________________

I Am Grateful For

Daily Meal Planner

MEAL PLAN		Macros Counts
Breakfast		Calories________ Carbs:________ Protein:______ Fats:__________
Mid Morning		Calories________ Carbs:________ Protein:______ Fats:__________
Lunch		Calories________ Carbs:________ Protein:______ Fats:__________
Afternoon		Calories________ Carbs:________ Protein:______ Fats:__________
Dinner		Calories________ Carbs:________ Protein:______ Fats:__________

	Calories	Carbs	Protein	Fats
Calculated Macros				
Daily Totals				

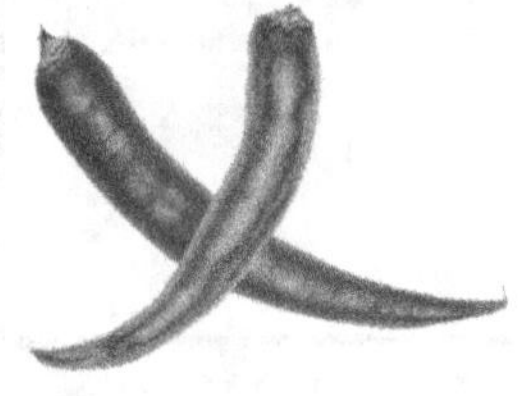
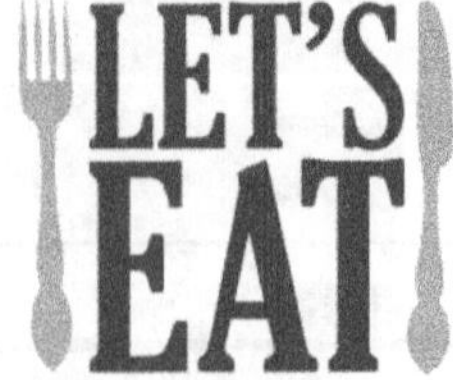

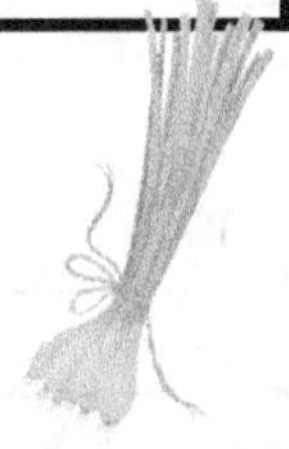

Daily Healthy Eating Habits

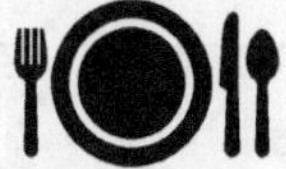 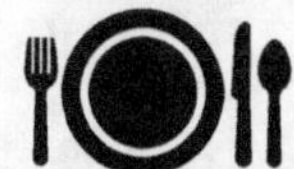

	Morning or Breakfast	Mid Day Or Lunch	Late Afternoon or Dinner	Evening Or Snacks
WATER- Drink 8-10 glasses or 3 L through out the day				
Veggies & Fruits- try to eat 5 servings each day				
Protein- Eat a palm size at each meal				
Healthy Fats- Eat fingertip - thumb size at each meal				
Follow Hand Portion Sizes at each meal				
Listen to Hunger & Fullness Cues				
Eat Mindfully & Slowly- Follow the 20 min meal				
Stop eating starchy carbs at 7pm				
Followed the 80/20 or 90/10 rule				
Any skipped meals				

Daily Exercise Plan

Activity	Length of W/O	Weight	Reps	Sets	Speed	Distance	Calories Burned

My Daily Reflections

Date:

Top 3 Daily Goals

- ☐ _______________________
- ☐ _______________________
- ☐ _______________________

My Action Steps To Help Me Reach My Daily Goals Are:

My Top 3 Strengths Are

- ☐ _______________________
- ☐ _______________________
- ☐ _______________________

Today I Found Happiness In

3 Things I Love About My Body

- ☐ _______________________
- ☐ _______________________
- ☐ _______________________

I Am Grateful For

Daily Meal Planner

MEAL PLAN		Macros Counts
Breakfast		Calories______ Carbs:______ Protein:______ Fats:________
Mid Morning		Calories______ Carbs:______ Protein:______ Fats:________
Lunch		Calories______ Carbs:______ Protein:______ Fats:________
Afternoon		Calories______ Carbs:______ Protein:______ Fats:________
Dinner		Calories______ Carbs:______ Protein:______ Fats:________

	Calories	Carbs	Protein	Fats
Calculated Macros				
Daily Totals				

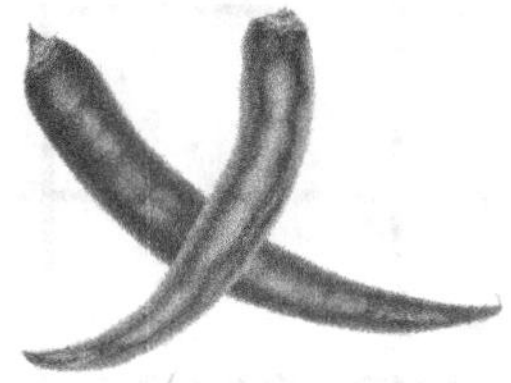

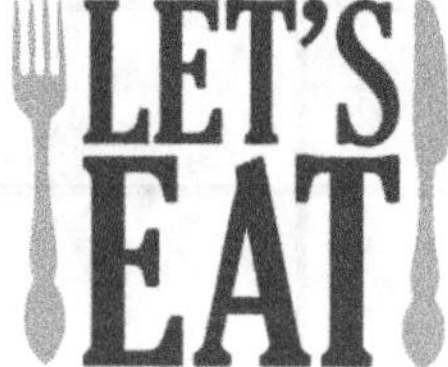

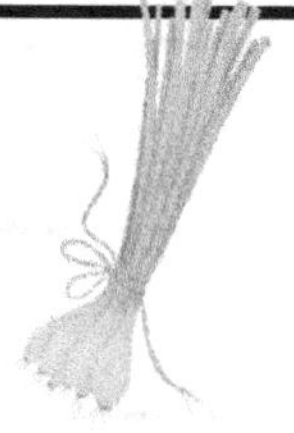

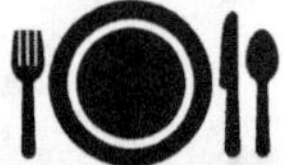 # Daily Healthy Eating Habits 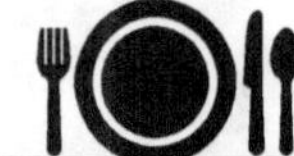

	Morning or Breakfast	Mid Day Or Lunch	Late Afternoon or Dinner	Evening Or Snacks
WATER- Drink 8-10 glasses or 3 L through out the day				
Veggies & Fruits- try to eat 5 servings each day				
Protein- Eat a palm size at each meal				
Healthy Fats- Eat fingertip - thumb size at each meal				
Follow Hand Portion Sizes at each meal				
Listen to Hunger & Fullness Cues				
Eat Mindfully & Slowly- Follow the 20 min meal				
Stop eating starchy carbs at 7pm				
Followed the 80/20 or 90/10 rule				
Any skipped meals				

Daily Exercise Plan

Activity	Length of W/O	Weight	Reps	Sets	Speed	Distance	Calories Burned

My Daily Reflections

Date:

⭐ Top 3 Daily Goals ⭐

- ☐ _______________________
- ☐ _______________________
- ☐ _______________________

My Action Steps To Help Me Reach My Daily Goals Are:

❤ My Top 3 Strengths Are ❤

- ☐ _______________________
- ☐ _______________________
- ☐ _______________________

Today I Found Happiness In

3 Things I Love About My Body

- ☐ _______________________
- ☐ _______________________
- ☐ _______________________

I Am Grateful For

Daily Meal Planner

MEAL PLAN		Macros Counts
Breakfast		Calories________ Carbs:________ Protein:________ Fats:__________
Mid Morning		Calories________ Carbs:________ Protein:________ Fats:__________
Lunch		Calories________ Carbs:________ Protein:________ Fats:__________
Afternoon		Calories________ Carbs:________ Protein:________ Fats:__________
Dinner		Calories________ Carbs:________ Protein:________ Fats:__________

	Calories	Carbs	Protein	Fats
Calculated Macros				
Daily Totals				

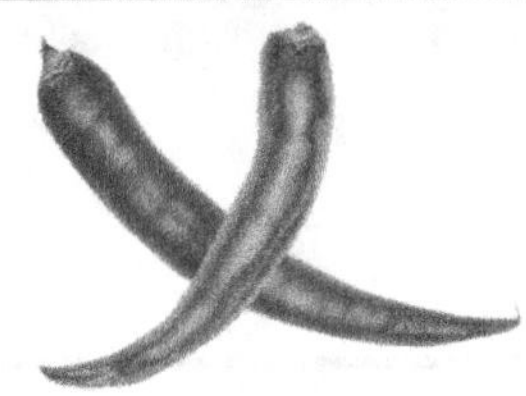

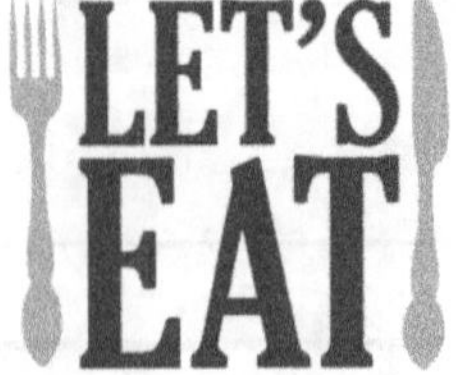

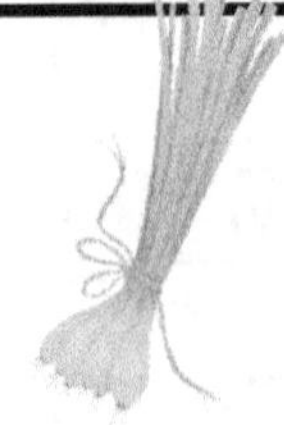

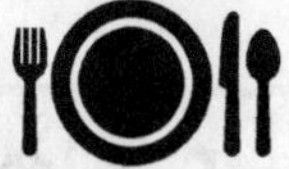 # Daily Healthy Eating Habits 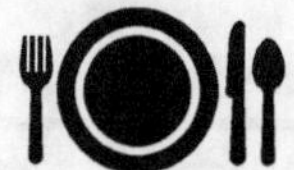

	Morning or Breakfast	Mid Day Or Lunch	Late Afternoon or Dinner	Evening Or Snacks
WATER- Drink 8-10 glasses or 3 L through out the day				
Veggies & Fruits- try to eat 5 servings each day				
Protein- Eat a palm size at each meal				
Healthy Fats- Eat fingertip - thumb size at each meal				
Follow Hand Portion Sizes at each meal				
Listen to Hunger & Fullness Cues				
Eat Mindfully & Slowly- Follow the 20 min meal				
Stop eating starchy carbs at 7pm				
Followed the 80/20 or 90/10 rule				
Any skipped meals				

Daily Exercise Plan

Activity	Length of W/O	Weight	Reps	Sets	Speed	Distance	Calories Burned

<table>
<tr><td>Week Of:</td><td>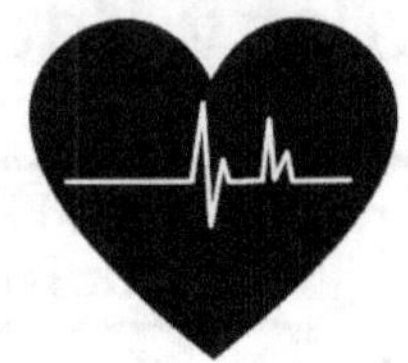</td><td>Track Your Blood Sugar</td></tr>
</table>

Date	Wake Up	Pre-Lunch	Afternoon	Pre-Dinner	Bedtime

Results

High					
Good					
Low					

Note Any Changes

CONGRATULATIONS! YOU DID IT!!

★★★★★★★★★★★★★★★★★★★★★★★

SPLURGE ON

SOMETHING

YOU'VE

WANTED

FOR

AGES

★★★★★★★★★★★★★★★★★★★★★★★

Thank you for purchasing The Weekly Meal Planner.

If you enjoyed this journal you may also enjoy some of my other journal:

Visit me at prevailhealthcoach.com to view my other health, wellness and fitness journals, kid's journals, colouring books and more!

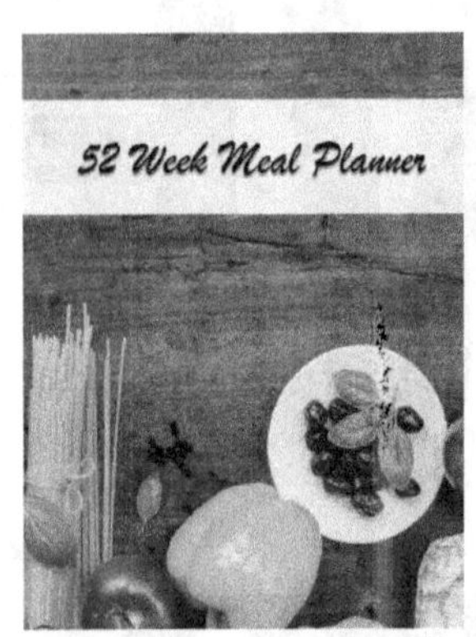

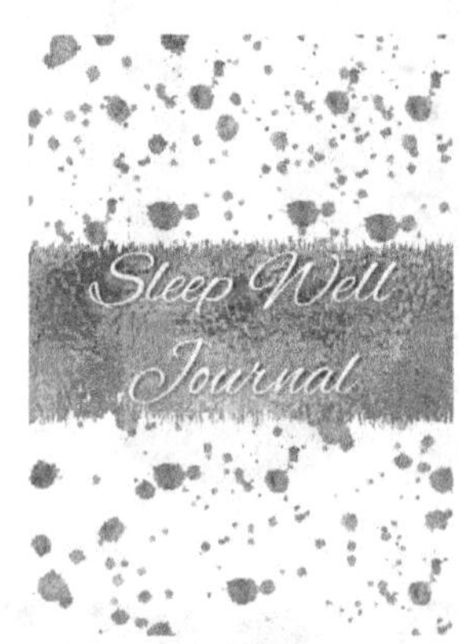

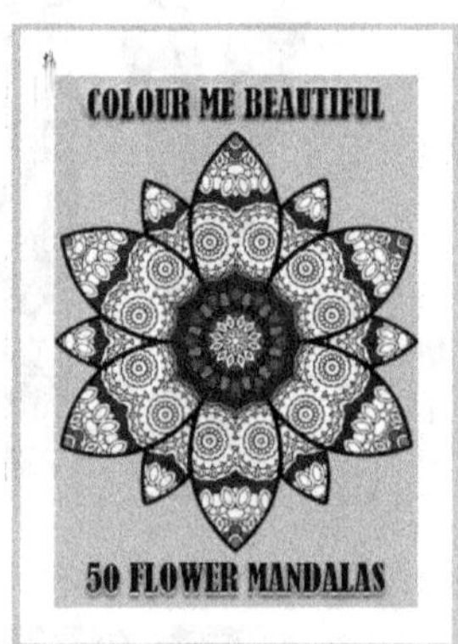

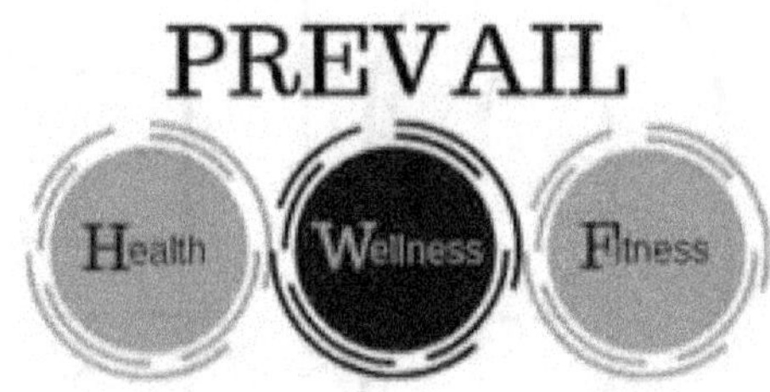